FROM ACUPRESSURE TO ZEN

FROM ACUPRESSURE TO ZEN

An Encyclopedia of Natural Therapies

BARBARA NASH

Hunter House

      Hunter House Inc., Publishers
      P.O. Box 2914
      Alameda, CA 94501-0914

LIBRARY OF CONGRESS CATALOGING-IN-PUBLICATION DATA

Nash, Barbara.
[A-Z of Complementary Health]
From Acupressure to Zen : an encyclopedia of natural therapies / Barbara Nash.
p. cm.
U.K. ed. published under the title: The A-Z of complementary health.
Includes bibliographical references.
ISBN 0-89793-190-4. — ISBN 0-89793-189-0 (pbk.)
1. Alternative medicine—Encyclopedias. 2. Self-care, Health—Encyclopedias.
3. Medicine, Popular—Encyclopedias. I. Title.
R733.N35 1995
615.5'03—dc20   95-33717

Project Editor: Lisa E. Lee
Production Manager: Paul J. Frindt
Cover design and illustration by Theresa Smith
Editors: Mali Apple, Lara Thompson
Proofreader: Susan Burckhard
Sales & Marketing: Corrine M. Sahli
Promotion & Publicity: Darcy Cohan
Administration: María Jesús Aguiló
Customer Support: Sarah Bhattacharjee, Joshua Tabisaura
Order Fulfillment: A & A Quality Shipping Services
Publisher: Kiran S. Rana

Typeset by 847 Communications, Alameda, CA
Printed and bound by Data Reproductions, Rochester Hills MI
Manufactured in the United States of America

9 8 7 6 5 4 3 2 1   First U.S. edition

ORDERING INFORMATION

Trade bookstores and wholesalers in the U.S. and Canada, please contact

PUBLISHERS GROUP WEST
4065 Hollis, Box 8843, Emeryville CA 94608
Telephone 1-800-788-3123 or (510) 658-3453
Fax (510) 658-1834

SPECIAL SALES

Hunter House books are available at special discounts when
purchased in bulk for sales promotions, premiums, or fundraising.
For details, please contact

Special Sales Department
HUNTER HOUSE INC.
P.O. Box 2914, Alameda CA 94501–0914
Telephone (510) 865-5282   Fax (510) 865-4295

COLLEGE TEXTBOOKS / COURSE ADOPTION ORDERS

Please contact Hunter House at the address and phone number above.

ORDERS BY INDIVIDUALS OR ORGANIZATIONS

Hunter House books are available through most bookstores
or can be ordered directly from the publisher by calling toll-free:

1-800-266-5592

To my brother Norman Henry,
whom I would so loved to have
benefited from this book.

LIST OF CONTENTS

PART TWO: A–Z of Common Conditions and Suitable Complementary Therapies

PART THREE: Complementary Therapies for Special Needs

NOTE TO THE READER

The material in this book is intended to provide an overview of the complementary approaches to health and well-being. Every effort has been made to provide accurate and dependable information. The reader should be aware that professionals in the field may have differing opinions and change is always taking place. Therefore, the author, publisher, and editors cannot be held responsible for any error, omission, or outdated material.

If you have any questions or concerns about the information in this book or the care and treatment of your self or your family, please consult a licensed health practitioner.

Some of the therapies, treatments, or products mentioned in this book have been trademarked. When the author and publisher were aware of a trademark claim, the designations have been printed with initial capital letters. The inclusion of a therapy, product, or organization in this book does not imply endorsement; omission does not imply criticism.

ACKNOWLEDGMENTS

The author and publishers would like to thank the following for their help in supplying information for this book but would like to stress that ultimately all opinions are those of the author.

Dr. Mark Yu, Academy of Chinese Acupuncture; Kate Kelly, The Society of Teachers of the Alexander Technique; Dr. Diane Waller, Goldsmiths' College, University of London; Peter Wesson, The Bury Clinic of Alternative Medicine; Dr. Malcolm Carruthers, Centre for Autogenic Training; Dr. Ela Shah; Judy Howard, The Dr. Edward Bach Centre; Angela Bradbury, Holistic Health College; Guy Gladstone, The Open Centre; Peter Staples, The Awakened Mind Ltd; Dr. David Bray, International Stress Management Association (U.K.); Matthew Bennett, British Chiropractic Association; Sheila Dainow, Skills with People; Danielle Melville, Craniosacral Therapy Association; Dr. Sir Peter Guy Manners, Bretforton Hall Clinic; Kay Kiernan, Bluestone Clinic; Barbara Traynor, ITA News; Jennifer Mackewn, Gestalt Psychotherapy Training Institute; Ian Stewart, Co-Director, Berne Institute; Heinz Zeylstra, The School of Phytotherapy; Sheilagh Creasy, The Institute for Complementary Medicine; Dr. Paul Barber, Department of Educational Studies, University of Surrey; Sue Washington, Centre Training School of Hypnotherapy and Psychotherapy; Wrio Russell, London School of Sports Massage; Monica Anthony; Dr. Ian Drysdale, British College of Naturopathy and Osteopathy; Penelope Robinson, The Chartered Society of Physiotherapy; Paul Guest, Polarity Therapy Association; Susan Cowan-Jenssen, The London Association of Primal Psychotherapists; Enid Eden, The Keys College of Radionics; Patricia Morrell, The Patricia Morrell Clinic and Teaching Centre; Jenny Crewdson, Certified Rolfer; Nicola Pooley, The Shiatsu

Society of Britain; John Harford, President, Nei Chia Association (G.B.); Valerie Brown, The Yoga Biomedical Trust; Gerry Smith, Tara Trust; Dr. Sandra Goodman; Dr. Robyn Young.

FOREWORD

To *complement* means to complete or to make whole. The complementary approach has gained in popularity because it helps many conditions previously labeled "incurable" or "chronic." Complementary medicine sees the symptom of an illness or condition as an outward sign of an imbalance between the physical, mental, and emotional levels and the vitality (spirit) of the patient, and attempts to reconcile all these factors. This concept involves a basic change of emphasis in our perception of the maintenance of good health. Most professional practitioners of complementary treatments feel that they complement the needs of the patient. They may also complement the work of orthodox doctors, an alliance in which both sides have an understanding and appreciation of the advantages the two forms of medicine offer.

The best advice for anyone wanting to try a complementary approach is to ask questions and to see which approach feels right. This will involve inquiring about all methods of treatment available and, where appropriate, talking to your doctor. Don't expect miracles, but on the other hand, don't persist with a treatment that seems to be having no effect. Although healing takes time, it should be possible to notice some reaction early on in the treatment. Healing is not just an absence of pain; it is also an increasing appreciation of all that life has to offer and an inner confidence that some personal control is being gained over illness or pain.

This book is an excellent general reference work on this complex subject and will serve to expand the knowledge and appreciation of complementary medicine for the increasing numbers of people who wish to try this approach.

Michael Endacott
The Institute for Complementary Medicine

PREFACE

Sooner or later anybody who moves in complementary therapy circles will hear the joke about the boss who is dashing off on vacation. Yelling over her shoulder at her secretary, she says: "One more thing. Cancel aromatherapy, psychotherapy, reflexology, osteopath, homoeopath, naturopath, crystal reading, Shiatsu, organic hairdresser. And see if I can be rebirthed next Thursday afternoon!"

Humor aside, the world of complementary therapies is a maze of rich possibilities, and the temptation to go in for several of them can be irresistible. Sometimes this does not matter. Many of them, in addition to complementing orthodox medical treatments, complement each other. At other times, it is wiser to entrust oneself to one pair of complementary hands and be guided by that practitioner. If another therapy is needed, you will be advised and, doubtless, passed on to another practitioner for safekeeping.

The first and most important consideration, whatever therapy you choose, is that you should choose a practitioner who is fully trained and qualified. At the moment it is still possible for people who are neither trained nor qualified to offer their services in some areas of complementary medicine. However gifted an unqualified "healer" might be, it is too much of a risk to entrust one's health to such a person.

Taking personal responsibility for one's health is not a self-indulgent fad—many of us spend more on servicing our cars than our bodies—it is a positive and life-enhancing step.

I have never doubted for one minute that most doctors do their utmost for their patients; but doctors who recognize the magic, wonder, and mystery of complementary therapies are very special doctors—the only kind I, and countless others, would wish to entrust ourselves and our loved ones to.

This book is written from a deep conviction that there are wonderful natural, health-enhancing and life-enhancing complementary remedies and therapies that will benefit each of us, whether we are coping with a common cold, a hiccup, or a life-threatening illness.

I hope and trust that this will be your experience, too.

Barbara Nash

INTRODUCTION

WHY COMPLEMENTARY THERAPIES?

The term *complementary therapy* has been used in this book in preference to *alternative therapy*. Some people have confined the use of the word *complementary* to treatments, such as massage and hydrotherapy, that *support* rather than *replace* orthodox forms of treatment. Here, however, the word is used to imply remedies and treatments that play both a supporting role and a replacing role.

The word *complement* also has the right connotations. There is a sense of balance, an inherent acceptance that both orthodox treatments *and* complementary therapy treatments have a part to play and that both must be allowed to play that part amicably and supportively. The use of the term *alternative* sometimes gives the impression that orthodox and alternative remedies and treatments are at odds with each other. There is an inherent air of disapproval, a lack of acceptance that benefits neither doctors nor patients.

Perhaps, like the word *complementary,* the use of the word *orthodox* needs some clarification. We all know what an orthodox person is—one who always behaves and dresses appropriately, conventionally. Likewise, we know what an unorthodox person is —one who is unconventional or unpredictable. The word *orthodox,* then, is associated with conventional, established, and proven. In the past, the word *alternative* was associated with "fringe," and taken to mean unorthodox and unproved. Today, the word *complementary* is understood to work within conventional medical disciplines.

This book begins from the premise that sometimes a decision must be made about whether to choose between orthodox or complementary treatment, but such a decision, whatever it is, need not imply criticism of either system.

ORTHODOX AND COMPLEMENTARY
THERAPIES TOGETHER

The opportunities for orthodox doctors and complementary practitioners to work together, as a team, for the benefit of themselves and their patients, have never been greater. This is confirmed daily by an increasing number of doctors, including both hospital and family doctors, qualifying in complementary therapies in addition to orthodox medical practices.

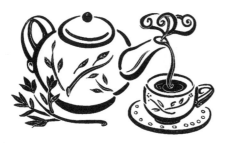

It is revealed in many other ways, too. Few orthodox doctors today would disagree with the emphasis that complementary practitioners place on the negative impacts of the following on physical, emotional, mental, and spiritual health: environmental factors, such as deforestation and global warming; lack of exercise; farming chemicals and insecticides; food additives—we are at the end of the chain; pollution—air, lead, noise, radiation, and water pollution; reaction to orthodox drug treatments, including overdependency and side effects; and social factors such as poverty, poor housing, and malnutrition.

Likewise, few orthodox doctors would disagree with an emphasis on the positive impact of complete (holistic) healing systems that place equal emphasis on body, emotion, mind, and spirit; eating for health and vitality; the need for exercise; and self-help measures to enhance and improve the physical, emotional, mental, and spiritual health and well-being.

Most family doctors would also be the first to admit that, with the best will in the world, the pressures of their work and people waiting to be seen often mean that they cannot spend all the time they would wish in discerning the underlying cause of a patient's anxiety, tension, and stress. Sometimes it simply has to be a prescription for a tranquilizer, rather than a counseling or psychotherapy session.

How much better, then, for the doctor to pause and ask: "Have you considered complementary therapy? I think you might find it much more beneficial in the long term than a short-term fix with this or that drug." There will, of course, always be patients who cannot afford the services of a complementary practitioner, but likewise there have always been, and hopefully always will be, complementary practitioners who do not refuse a patient for financial reasons.

Two undisputed advantages of complementary therapies are that the practitioner has more time to devote to you and your problem than most doctors have, and the waiting room is rarely as full as a family doctor's waiting room. Even when it is busy, appointments usually run on time.

One of the funniest experiences I ever had in complementary therapy was when I was waiting to see an osteopath. Apart from me, there was only a dachshund, lying patiently, head on paws. Oh, good, I thought, even though I am early, I will be next. Imagine my astonishment when the osteopath's voice boomed out, "Muffin," and the dog staggered to its feet, followed by its mistress. Later, Muffin's mistress explained that the dog hurt his back jumping a low wall to flirt with a passing friend. He was paralyzed, and had to be carried in a sling. Thanks to the osteopath, he was walking again. Later, I heard that the osteopath had treated a number of animals, including race horses. Every time I went, I peeped through the waiting room window to see who—or what—was in front of me!

THE PLACEBO EFFECT

My reaction to the suggestion that complementary therapies are only a placebo has always been, so what? There may be—most likely is—some truth in the assertion that some complementary therapies have a placebo effect and that with or without them the result would be the same. The point, surely, is that the person *feels* better, which is more important than how or why.

It is equally true that not all the successes can be attributed to the feel-good factor. Like it or not—and some people do not, whatever the conviction and personal testimony of others—many remedies and treatments work at non-placebo levels.

MAGIC OR MIRACLE CURE?

The cure may be neither magical nor miraculous; the important thing is to accept that remarkable healing has been known to take place. Some can be explained in satisfactory scientific terms; some cannot and perhaps never will be. While this is frustrating for people who want an answer for everything, I am often reminded of this saying: "For those who believe in the miraculous, no explanation is necessary. For those who do not believe, no explanation is possible."

Having said that, it is important not to expect a magic or miracle cure; if you do, you may be disappointed. Sometimes recovery is slow; sometimes recovery is impossible. Sometimes only symptoms can be alleviated, and compassion and understanding and pain relief offered. But for the person bearing the symptoms and pain, the "only" is wonderful and miraculous in its own way.

WHAT TO EXPECT

Some complementary therapies achieve a dramatic and impressive result in a short time, with the additional bonus of long-term relief; others do not. Some may never offer an improvement, let alone a remedy or a cure.

The majority of practitioners—like the majority of doctors—are essentially honest, honorable, and responsible people whose integrity can be taken for granted. Having said that, there are always exceptions, and where there is money to be made, there are those who will. make it without really earning it.

It is always a personal decision, but if a therapy is not having the desired effect, if your condition is at the least not improving and at the worst deteriorating, think again. It is true that some conditions get worse before they get better, but if this remains the case for longer than appears to be natural or normal, return to your doctor and reconsider the approach. Nothing comes cheap, and willing a remedy to hurry up and work may not be the answer and may delay you from finding something else that will.

WHY NOT ACUPUNCTURE OR IRIDOLOGY OR...?

When you are considering the various therapies in Part One and the conditions for which they are recommended in Part Two, you may wonder why a particular therapy is not included under an ailment that you know has been eased by a particular treatment. Such a list can never be fully comprehensive. For the purposes of this book, specific therapies have been linked to specific conditions and diseases because they are the ones for which success is most often claimed. There are doubtless other successes— something that is recommended for this may also alleviate that. If this happens to you, tell your practitioner and broadcast it to whomever needs to know.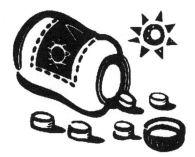

WHAT DOCTORS THINK

People are sometimes puzzled that their family doctor looks so blank when the possibility of trying a complementary therapy is mentioned, or the doctor's advice is sought, as is recommended so often in this book. Remember that the doctor may not have sufficient knowledge of a particular therapy to approve or disapprove, recommend or not. Given what family doctors must know and the constant updating of knowledge in the field of conventional medicine, let alone the constant flow of new information about complementary treatments, that is fair enough. He or she can always ask for time to consider, think about your request, and then make the necessary inquiries from likely sources after you have left.

Throughout Part One, the sections entitled "What doctors think" will give you some idea of the doubts, fears, and resistance that you may meet when consulting orthodox family doctors and hospital doctors and consultants. Although some of these doubts may stem from closed minds and biased attitudes, many of their fears and resistances might be perfectly justifiable.

GETTING INTO THE SPIRIT

One aspect of some complementary therapies that is often initially overlooked by those who seek them, and sometimes not mentioned in the early stages by those who practice them, is that many are based on religious beliefs and practices, and some actually stem from religious disciplines. Meditation, yoga, Zen, and Zen garden therapy, for example, are as much a part of the religious practices of the Buddhist and Hindu religions as prayer is of Christianity. As it is not unknown for people who have taken up a complementary therapy to also take up the religion that is behind it, a brief explanation of some relevant eastern religions is included in this book (see page 225).

THE APPEAL OF COMPLEMENTARY THERAPIES

Complementary therapies are drawing people in unprecedented numbers. Two main reasons are behind this: the attraction of the complementary therapies themselves, and a dissatisfaction with orthodox medicine, particularly the unpleasant side effects of some drug treatments.

The attraction of complementary therapies often includes the emphasis that is placed on health rather than on illness, on prevention as well as cure. People are also attracted by the emphasis on self-healing life-forces, which can be rallied, rebalanced, and remarshaled in times of health threats and troubles; and the emphasis placed on "natural," an evocative word that many people associate with concepts such as wholesome, nourishing, and inherently good.

Others are drawn by the emphasis that is placed on "traditional." This is, perhaps, the most surprising, but many people associate traditional with complementary because they sense—as is true—that many of the remedies precede or predate orthodox medicine's remedies. Consider, for example, the case of the Chinese traditional medicine doctor and four children suffering from eczema. Doctors at Great Ormond Street Children's Hospital in London were astonished when they were told that extraordinary improvements in the children were achieved by a traditional Chinese concoction of twelve herbs made into a tea.

There is also the appeal of being adventurous, of seeking out the unknown and unusual—the mysterious pulling power of the east, of Chinese and Indian remedies as opposed to western. Finally, there is the welcome—the feeling that one is valued and worthy of another's time, interest, and compassion. There is nothing more comforting than being the center of attention, if only for thirty minutes of your practitioner's day; nothing more interesting than being told something unusual about yourself, something you have never heard before, such as, "Today, your aura is blue-green . . . gold-green"; nothing more relieving than receiving a finger-thumb-hand jolt to the spine that unlocks years of pain. This is the stuff that dreams are made of—this is healing. Read on!

PART ONE

A–Z of Complementary Therapies

ACUPRESSURE

Origins   This massage healing technique has been practiced for over three thousand years in China and Japan and is used today in most countries of the world.

What it is   A combination of massage and acupuncture, acupressure involves the use of the practitioner's thumbs and fingertips (and sometimes the palms, knees, elbows, and feet) to apply firm pressure massage on the same pressure points along the body's energy paths, or meridians, used in acupuncture. The meridians, a network of energy channels, influence the major organs of the body. According to the pressure points used and the amount of pressure applied, acupressure is also known as Shin Tao, Jin Shin Do, and Shiatsu.

At your first session, the practitioner will first note your medical history and discuss such things as diet and lifestyle. You will be asked to sit or lie down on the floor or a table, and the fingertip pressure massage will begin. It is advisable to wear loose clothing for acupressure sessions, which usually last about thirty minutes.

The practitioner may also teach you some safe self-help acupressure methods to use at home, advise you on your eating habits, and suggest other alternative therapies to assist you with existing disorders.

What it is used for   Acupressure balances the flow of energy, enhances natural vitality, and promotes maintenance of health and self-healing. It is believed to prevent illness and to relieve existing ailments, such as digestive problems, and painful symptoms, such as arthritis. It is used mainly to complement other alternative therapies, such as naturopathy.

It is used for treating arthritis; back pain; catarrh; claustrophobia; colds; colitis; dizziness; eyestrain; fainting; frozen shoulder; gout; indigestion; irritable bowel syndrome; joint problems; kidney complaints; laryngitis; lumbago; migraines; nausea and vomiting; neuralgia; pain; phobias; prolapse; ringing in the ears; sciatica; slipped disc; sports injuries; stammering; sweating; teeth grinding; tiredness; travel sickness; and vertigo.

What doctors think

There has not been sufficient scientific research for doctors to feel entirely at ease about the claims that are made about the benefits of acupressure. Some doctors, however, have been reassured by research that shows that people who wear an acupressure band, often called a "sea band," on their wrists are often unaffected by habitual travel sickness and nausea related to pregnancy and general anesthetics.

Warning

Persistent pain is the body's alarm system and should be discussed with your family doctor. Always consult your doctor before using acupressure for anything but ailments you would normally treat at home.

Some acupressure treatments are not suitable for pregnant women. Your practitioner should advise you regarding this.

ACUPUNCTURE

Origins

This ancient therapy, which uses needles to treat common ailments and diseases, has been practiced in China for about five thousand years. Its use is associated with the idea that the stimulation of specific areas under or deep inside the skin affects how certain organs of the body function.

What it is

Traditional acupuncture is based on the principle that good health depends on the balanced functioning of the body's motivating energy, or Qi (pronounced "chee"). Qi flows throughout the body, but is concentrated in channels in the tissues of the body, known as meridians. Fourteen main meridians run from the hands and feet to the body and head.

Acupuncture, meaning "to prick with a needle," is the art of expertly and painlessly piercing the skin with disposable needles at different puncture points along the meridians. There are almost a thousand puncture points.

The aim of acupuncture is to maintain health and to restore the balance among the physical, emotional, mental, and spiritual aspects of the individual—particularly the balance between the equal and opposite qualities of Qi, namely the yin (passive) and the yang (stimulating). In the theory of Chinese medicine, many factors are believed to upset this balance, to disturb the flow of Qi, and to cause disharmony and ill health. These factors include emotional states, such as anxiety, fear, grief, and stress; undereating or

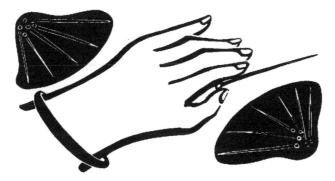

overeating; drugs, both illicit and prescribed; environmental and occupational conditions; weather conditions; hereditary factors; infections; and shock and trauma.

Acupuncture is believed to bring about restoration of yin-yang balance, helping the person attain a natural state of harmony.

During the first session, the practitioner notes the person's medical history, diet, and lifestyle, takes the pulse, and aims to determine—by questions, answers, and observation—the nature of the existing disharmony. Having decided on the cause or causes of the problem, the appropriate puncture points and method of treatment are selected.

Acupuncture needles are so fine that in the hands of skilled practitioners there is little discomfort when they are inserted into the skin. A tingle, known as the needle sensation, may be felt while the needle is in place. During the treatment, the needles are either withdrawn immediately or left in place for several minutes.

Many people experience a feeling of peace and relaxation during the treatment.

Treatments are usually given once or twice a week. Some people need only a couple of treatments; others need treatment for several months.

What it is used for

Acupuncture's best-known use is for easing and relieving the pain of ailments such as arthritis, back problems, and rheumatism. It is also increasingly used to treat addictions such as smoking.

Success has been claimed for treating acid stomach; addiction; agoraphobia; allergies; angina; anorexia; anxiety; arthritis; asthma; back pain; blood pressure (high and low); bronchitis; bunions; catarrh; pain during childbirth; chronic fatigue syndrome; colitis; coughs; depression; eczema; emphysema; fatigue; fluid retention; gallstones; gout; hay fever; headaches; hip complaints; indigestion; infertility; insomnia; irritable bowel syndrome; joint problems; kidney complaints; lumbago; menopausal problems; menstrual problems; migraines; mood swings; neck pain; nervous disorders; neuralgia; obesity; panic attacks; pain; postnatal depression; premenstrual tension; prostate problems; rheumatism; ringing in the ears; sexual problems; sciatica; shingles; shock and trauma; sinus problems; weight loss; slipped disc; smoking; sports injuries; stress; teeth grinding; tension; thyroid disorders; tooth and gum disorders; travel sickness; ulcers (gastric, duodenal, and leg); vertigo; warts; water retention; and wheezing.

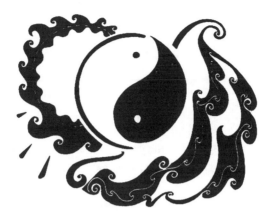

What doctors think
While there is a general acceptance among western doctors that what they call "trigger points" exist some distance from affected or diseased organs and that their stimulation can relieve pain, many continue to await scientific confirmation of the various claims before committing themselves to acupuncture. Others express concern that patients ignore what their symptoms and pain are trying to tell them and thus delay seeking vital medical treatment.

Warning
Qualified acupuncturists observe a strict code of practice, including guidelines on hygiene and medically approved needles. Do not consult anybody who is not fully qualified.

Anybody may claim to be an acupuncturist, so it is important to confirm that your acupuncturist is licensed by the National Commission for the Certification of Acupuncturists.

ALEXANDER TECHNIQUE

Origins

This now greatly respected technique came into being when Australian actor Frederick Mathis Alexander discovered that many health problems could be alleviated by a simple improvement of posture in movement. He believed that good posture or good use of the self enhances health and well-being; bad posture or bad use of the self diminishes them.

He introduced his method, which later became known as the Alexander technique, to London in 1904, and it became instantly popular with actors. He continued his work in the United States, achieving international acclaim and fame before his death in 1955.

What it is

The Alexander technique retrains the way we use our bodies by teaching us how to recognize harmful habitual movement patterns and how to use the muscles of the body with minimum effort and maximum efficiency. Attention is given to such movements as getting in and out of a chair, sitting, standing, walking, and working at a variety of work surfaces.

The lessons usually consist of a course of about thirty sessions, which last thirty to forty-five minutes. After this, you are usually considered ready to continue refining the technique on your own.

The teacher begins by studying how you use your body when sitting, standing, walking, and so on. He or she notes any inappropriate muscular tension—created by such things as holding the head or shoulders incorrectly—that throws the rest of the body off balance and out of alignment. Poor habitual posture is changed by instruction and gentle manipulation. The new alignment may feel unnatural at first because the bad habit, long practiced, feels natural. Given time and patience, however—yours and the teacher's—the posture and movement of the body will improve.

What it is used for

By correcting habitual bad posture, the Alexander technique alleviates health-threatening tensions and enables the muscles to work in a harmonious, more efficient way.

The resulting good posture benefits the whole person and can change our perception of ourselves and how we are living our lives. Breathing is also improved, making the Alexander technique of particular benefit to asthma sufferers. Pain in the lower back and discomforts in the elderly—frequently due to habitual misuse—are also lessened.

The Alexander technique has been used to alleviate anxiety; asthma; back pain (lower); blood pressure (high); chronic fatigue syndrome; colitis; depression; exhaustion; headaches; irritable bowel syndrome; lumbago; menstrual problems; mood swings; muscular tension; neck pain; nervous disorders; osteoarthritis; panic attacks; postnatal depression; respiratory disorders; rheumatoid arthritis; sciatica; snoring; sports injuries; stress; tension; ulcers; varicose veins; and wheezing.

What doctors think   Recent scientific research has supported beliefs about the connection between poor posture and one's state of mind, so most doctors are positive about the Alexander technique. Many, however, do not recommend the technique simply because they have not heard of it or do not know enough about it.

AROMATHERAPY

Origins   An ancient art, aromatherapy is mentioned in the writings of the earliest civilizations— Mesopotamian, Egyptian, Indian, and Chinese—and the first evidence of distilled pure essences was recorded in the eleventh century in Europe. The modern concept of aromatherapy was developed by Marguerite Maury, an Austrian biochemist, in the middle of the twentieth century. It was used by René Gattefosse during World War I to treat wounded soldiers. A chemist, Gattefosse claimed that, in addition to healing, the fragrances masked the odor of soldiers' gangrenous wounds and that proximity to the fragrance of pine protected soldiers from respiratory disorders. Not surprisingly, Swiss sanitoriums were usually sited by pine forests.

What it is   Aromatherapy is the treating of common ailments and health problems with highly concentrated oils that have been extracted from plants and trees. The aromatic essences are believed to contain medicinal properties and a natural healing power. They are often used in massage, but can also be ingested, inhaled, used on compresses, or added to hand and foot baths or to bath water.

Aromatherapists use up to 130 different oils, which they divide into three main categories: (1) invigorating, refreshing, and uplifting oils—for example, rosemary; (2) oils for regulating and toning up the body—for example, lemon grass; (3) oils that relax and soothe—for example, orange blossom.

Aromatic plant essences and oils can be used for beauty, healing, or simply for pleasure. They can be blended into vegetable oils and creams for skin-care preparations, added to bath water, used in steam inhalations for treating colds and flu symptoms, used for massage, and heated as mood-enhancing room perfumers.

Aromatherapy involves the mechanisms of olfaction (the smelling of aromas) and skin

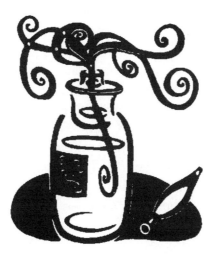

absorption (the entering of aromas into the body through the skin), and the influence of aromas on the nervous system.

Aromatherapy is regarded as especially successful for the treatment of recurring illnesses, nervous and stress-related disorders, and for patients who are suffering from side effects of drugs used in orthodox medicine.

At your first session with an aromatherapist, you will be asked about your general health and lifestyle, including diet. Oils will then be selected and mixed based on what you have told the therapist and what the therapist has observed.

Aromatherapy massage treatment lasts about thirty minutes for a partial massage, ninety minutes for a full-body massage.

Courses that teach the basics of aromatherapy, and how to use the oils that have been specially selected for you on a self-help basis at home, are available.

What it is used for

Aromatherapy is used in the treatment of agoraphobia; anemia; anal problems; anger; anxiety; arthritis; asthma; blisters; blood pressure (high and low); bladder problems; boils; bronchitis; bruises; bunions; burns; bursitis; catarrh; chapping; chicken pox; chronic fatigue syndrome; circulation problems; colds; colic; coughs; cramps; croup; cystitis; dandruff; depression; diarrhea; eczema; emphysema; flatulence; foot problems; frozen shoulder; fungal infections; genital herpes; headaches; hemorrhoids; indigestion; insomnia; manic-depressive illness; menopausal problems;

menstrual problems; mood swings; nervous disorders; neuralgia; nose and throat ailments; pain; panic attacks; phobias; pimples; postnatal depression; premenstrual tension; psoriasis; scalds; sexual problems; shingles; shock and trauma; sinus problems; sleep disorders; sneezing; sports injuries; stress; sweating; tension; thrush; tiredness; travel sickness; and warts.

What doctors think

Aromatherapy is now offered as an additional therapy in some hospitals, and scientific research is currently being carried out worldwide. Though the claims for its many benefits remain to be substantiated to all doctors' satisfaction, an increasing number are positive about its therapeutic uses.

Warning

Use essences with care, on the advice of a qualified aromatherapist. Do not apply undiluted oils directly to the skin. They can damage the skin or cause allergic reactions. Essences should not be swallowed unless they are diluted and then only if they are supplied by and used under the supervision of a trained aromatherapist.

For purposes other than massage, always buy pure, undiluted essential oils. For massage, use oils diluted in vegetable oil, almond oil, or alcohol. Many practitioners prefer organically grown oils, which eliminates possible nerve damage from organophosphates.

ART THERAPY

Origins

Art therapy was first developed in Britain in the 1940s, mainly through the work of artist Adrian Hill, psychotherapist Irene Champernowne, and the postwar rehabilitation movements.

What it is

Now a popular therapy worldwide, it is used as an alternative to, or enhancement of, traditional psychiatric treatment, to help people find relief by expressing themselves through drawing, painting, and other art media. Sir Winston Churchill, for example, turned to art when suffering from an overload of stress and tension brought about by the affairs of state.

Art therapists practice in clinics, hospitals, and special schools, and in private practice, and see people both on an individual and a group-session basis. They are good listeners who, in addition to art training and qualifications, are trained in art therapy at the postgraduate level, enabling them to appreciate the needs of people

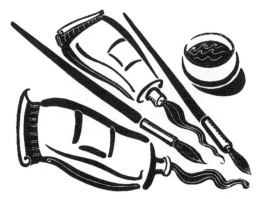

who have serious communication problems or emotional and psychological disturbances.

With new patients, they usually begin with the reassurance that nobody has to be "good at art" to enjoy its benefits. The most important aspect of art therapy is self-expression—in whatever form that takes, using whatever materials are available. The results, once the patient has overcome initial resistance to working in front of a stranger or strangers, can be astonishing. When inhibitions are lessened, the images that emerge can be powerfully evocative for both patient and therapist. So much that has been contained, submerged, or repressed—with harmful consequences—can now be released, allowing patient and therapist to resolve the problems together.

Art therapy is an ongoing process in which patients are encouraged to continue to express themselves through art, collages, and crafts at home.

What it is used for

Art therapy is used primarily for children or adults who are emotionally or psychologically disturbed, hospitalized on a long-term or acute basis, or have physical or learning disabilities.

Group art therapy is particularly recommended for people who have withdrawn from everyday life and contacts, and for those who have great difficulty relating to others. It is also considered therapeutic for people suffering from anorexia nervosa; bereavement; bulimia; low self-esteem; physical or learning difficulties; stress, and tension.

What doctors think   Most people first see an art therapist on the recommendation of a medical practitioner. As a result of research, personal experience, and the fact that it is now a profession in the health services and social sciences, doctors usually give it their blessing as a valid method.

AURA THERAPY

Origins   The aura is an ancient concept, portrayed as golden halos in early Christian art and as areas of light in eastern sculpture, Aboriginal paintings, and on Native American totem poles.

What it is   Every person, animal, and plant is said to have a visible aura, often described as magnetic field. Aura therapists believe that certain auras are harmonious—explaining why we feel peaceful in

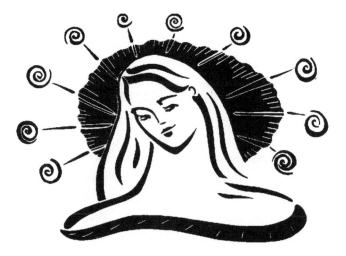

certain places and with certain people—while other auras conflict and produce less positive results. Auras are also claimed to indicate a person's state of health, emotion, mind, and spirit and to reveal their vulnerabilities.

The nine main colors of the aura are black/gray, blue, green, indigo, orange, red, yellow, violet, and white. Each color is thought to reveal aspects of a person's physical, emotional, mental, and spiritual states.

Practitioners are usually faith healers or practice other forms of complementary therapies. There are no special qualifications, other than an ability to see auras and to use the knowledge to fight disease. Some people believe, however, that only gifted psychics can do this.

Contact with a practitioner is usually made through other therapies, such as homeopathy, naturopathy, or faith healing. The therapist usually begins by observing the person's aura. A dull aura, for example, could indicate the existence of health problems; soft, vulnerability to events and other people; hard, insecurity; or green, mental versatility. Treatment may take the form of using his or her own energy—aura—to make healing spiritual adjustments to the other person's aura.

What it is used for

An awareness of auras enables a person to be more perceptive and more sensitive to people and surroundings. In a spiritual sense, a person is enabled to be in tune with subtle universal forces, from which life-enhancing energy and power can be drawn.

Aura therapy seeks to establish a person's physical, mental, and emotional states, reveal disorders and diseases of bodily parts and organs, and highlight general tensions and stress-related problems.

It is considered particularly helpful for people who have a desire to be more aware of themselves, of others, and of creation, and to develop spiritually.

What doctors think   Some doctors, having substituted the words *energy emissions* for *aura*, accept the possibility that such things can alert us to the presence of disease. Most await scientific findings on whether or not auras, even if they exist, can be sufficiently understood and diagnosed to help with disease.

AURICULAR THERAPY

Origins   This therapy was practiced in ancient China, Greece, and Egypt, and for at least four centuries in Mediterranean countries. It was rediscovered in the 1950s by a French man, Dr. Paul Nogier, who started to seek proof that acupuncture needle points on the ear could act as a reflection of the state of the whole human body.

What it is   The therapy consists of "needling" the ear, which is said to have over two hundred acupuncture pressure points that are related to the whole human body. Auricular therapists claim that waves of healing are sent to whatever part of the body is unwell.

Before offering auricular therapy, the practitioner will note your medical history, hereditary factors, lifestyle, and diet. The ears are then examined for deformities and marks, including warts, nodules, and skin texture. For a serious illness, the therapist may want to see a person on a daily basis for two or three days; once a week is more common for ordinary ailments.

The therapist locates the area to be treated either by running a probe over the ear until an area of discomfort is located, or by passing a pencil-shaped electrode over the ear and observing any abnormalities recorded on a meter. Having determined the problem, the therapist begins the treatment.

A self-help procedure is sometimes offered to people who find it difficult to attend regular sessions. For this, the therapist inserts semipermanent needles, which resemble tiny thumbtacks. These are left in for several days, and the patient simply presses the needles every hour or—for people who are trying to alleviate a particular addiction—every time he or she feels an urge to indulge in the addiction.

What it is used for

Auricular therapy has been used to treat addiction (including alcohol, food, drugs, and smoking); anorexia; arthritis; asthma; gout; indigestion; migraines; nervous problems; pain control (in childbirth, at the dentist, and pre- and post-surgery for minor and major operations); panic attacks; urinary disorders; and wheezing.

What doctors think   Unless your doctor specializes in Chinese therapies, you may not be encouraged to use this complementary therapy. Most doctors remain uneasy about it, despite the fact that it has been widely practiced, with good results, for decades in China.

AUTOGENIC TRAINING THERAPY

Origins   German neurologist Johann Schultz, who was very aware of the beneficial effects of using hypnotism on his patients, developed autogenic training therapy in the 1920s.

What it is   A self-healing form of profound relaxation, autogenic therapy consists of six mental exercises. The exercises focus in turn on relaxing sensations of heaviness and warmth in the arms and legs; a regular heartbeat; a natural pattern of breathing; abdominal warmth; cooling of the forehead; and "intentional exercises," which, as the name suggests, have the intention of relieving suppressed tension, sadness, and anger. The six exercises are designed to relieve stress and help self-healing through deep relaxation; they also promote general health and well-being and the prevention and cure of a variety of mental and physical health problems. They are carried out with the eyes shut, sitting or lying in a comfortable, stable position.

The practitioner usually teaches the therapy to groups of about six people on a weekly basis. The course lasts about two months, and each session begins with a group sharing of how the week went and how each person responded to the exercises.

The phrase *autogenic discharges* refers to sensations or muscle movements that accompany the release of stored tensions.

What it is used for

Autogenic therapy is used for a host of ailments, including addictions; anxiety; back pain; bronchitis; chronic fatigue syndrome; colitis; cramps; depression; eczema; frozen shoulder; hemorrhoids; indigestion; insomnia; irritable bowel syndrome; jet lag; lumbago; migraines; mood swings; nervous disorders; panic attacks; postnatal depression; sciatica; shock and trauma; sports injuries; stress; tension; and ulcers.

It is also claimed to improve the performance of athletes and dancers and help them recover more quickly from their exertions. Business people use autogenic therapy to relieve stress.

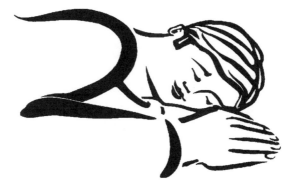

Practitioners also use the intentional exercises to help people who have repressed negative emotions, such as anger, resentment, and jealousy.

What doctors think

There is a wealth of scientific evidence to back up the benefits of autogenic training and therapy, and it is available in many hospitals and through private medical practices. Doctors often recommend it as a complementary therapy.

AUTOSUGGESTION THERAPY

Origins

Emile Coué, a French apothecary, initiated this theory of self-healing by hypnosis in the 1890s, when he became convinced that people could "will" recovery by imagining themselves healed or well.

What it is

Sometimes known as Couéism, autosuggestion is a hypnotherapy technique similar to meditation. However, instead of repeating a mantra, the person is taught to empty his or her mind of other thoughts and distractions and then to repeat certain positive phrases, silently or aloud. For example, the maxim for which Coué is most famous is, "Every day in every way, I am getting better and better." Coué believed that the repetition of such maxims, usually repeated twenty times at each occasion, has a positive effect on the body and mind by influencing a person at both the conscious and unconscious level.

The method is practiced night and morning, preferably just before falling asleep and just after awaking. Great emphasis is placed on regularity, the idea being that the autosuggestion weakens if neglected. Meditation (see page 100) is regarded as complementary to this therapy.

The technique is now used by practitioners of other complementary therapies, such as autogenic training and therapy (see page 28) and visualization therapy (see page 137).

It is not recommended for people who are against hypnotism, as their resistance will be counterproductive.

What it is used for   Autosuggestion therapy is used in the treatment of addiction (food, alcohol and drugs, and smoking); allergies; asthma; depression; mood swings; nervous disorders; pain (for example, during childbirth); panic attacks; phobias; psychosomatic illnesses; postnatal depression; shock and trauma; stress; and tension.

What doctors think   The medical profession was aggressively critical of the theory when it was first introduced. Since then, attitudes have softened, and doctors now accept that autosuggestion can influence a person physically and mentally. They warn, however, that it should not be used instead of or to replace orthodox treatments for serious illnesses and diseases from which a patient is unlikely to recover, or for people who are emotionally or mentally unstable.

Warning   Autosuggestion therapy should be used only by people of sound mind. It is considered unsuitable for people who have a history of emotional or mental disorders, and may even worsen the condition of people suffering from psychotic disorders by taking them still further from reality. Consult your family doctor before beginning this therapy.

AVERSION THERAPY

See Behavioral Therapy

AYURVEDIC MEDICINES

Origins   An ancient Indian holistic medicine system (its name means "science of life"), ayurvedic medicine places equal emphasis on treating the body, emotions, mind, and spirit. It covers many branches of nonorthodox medicine.

What it is   It remains an important medicine system in India, especially in rural areas. Its increasing popularity in the west stems from the fact that many westerners are disillusioned with the prescription-oriented approach of conventional medicine and are increasingly receptive to holistic systems that place a greater emphasis on prevention than on cure and healing.

In the ayurvedic system, everything and everybody is said to embody three basic life forces, or elements, which control all physical and mental processes: *kapha* (pronounced *kaph*), moon force; *pitta* (pronounced *pit*), sun force; and *vata* (pronounced *vat*), wind force. When *kapha*, *pitta,* and *vata* are in balance in an individual, good health results; when there is an imbalance, poor health results. Ayurvedic practitioners use the *kapha, pitta,* and *vata* principles to better understand their patients' current state of body, emotions, mind, and spirit, and to determine what is lacking and needed to attain better all-around health.

The ayurvedic treatments are of three main types, dietary, medicinal, and practical. They are used for four main categories of conditions: accidental, mental, natural (which includes childbirth and aging), and physical ailments.

Dietary advice usually recommends fresh food, eaten *slowly* in its natural season, in a calm frame of mind and tranquil surroundings. Fasting is sometimes recommended.

Medicinal remedies are primarily naturopathic, including eight thousand herbal, mineral, and vegetable medicines for prevention and treatment. Homeopathic and orthodox drugs are sometimes prescribed.

Practical aids consist of such things as breathing exercises, counseling, enemas, meditation, and yoga.

When you consult an ayurvedic doctor, the practitioner will first ask about your medical history, diet, and general lifestyle; take your pulse; and note the condition of your skin, eyes, nails, and tongue. As in all holistic therapies, your physical, emotional, mental, and spiritual states are taken into account before treatment begins. Patients are encouraged to keep in regular touch with the practitioner, so that

therapy can be applied on a preventive, as well
as a cure, basis.

**What it is
used for**

Ayurvedic therapy will, it is claimed, benefit
everybody, including those who are not ill.
Success is particularly claimed for a multitude of
common ailments, illnesses, and diseases,
including arthritis; asthma; depression; eczema;
indigestion; and stress.

**What doctors
think**

This holistic approach is generally accepted.

BACH FLOWER REMEDIES

Origins

These remedies are named after Edward Bach,
an orthodox British doctor, who, in the course of
his medical career, became committed to the
belief that natural plant cures exist for every
human ailment. Dr. Bach and others who use his
remedies believe that illness is caused by an
inner imbalance, and that nature provides
healing remedies to correct this imbalance.

The Bach remedies were first prepared from
the dew that collects on flowers and later
produced in greater quantities by floating freshly
picked flowers on spring water, in the sunshine.

**What they
are**

The thirty-eight Bach remedies are formulated to
treat the whole person, rather than just symptoms
or ailments. They are chosen primarily for mood
and psychological outlook, because the therapy is
based on the theory that correction of emotional

imbalance is the key to improved health. In this way, the Bach remedies may complement orthodox treatment for physical ailments, shock, and trauma. Very much a self-awareness, self-help system, the use of the remedies is not dependent on counselors or practitioners. Each person is asked to attempt an honest appraisal of his or her attitudes, habits, emotional, mental, and physical states, general personality, and approach to life.

Having decided the "type" of person you are—for example, apathetic, apprehensive, fearful, impatient, indecisive, irritable, jealous—you select the appropriate remedy or remedies to correct the health-threatening imbalance.

There is a professional register of qualified Bach flower remedy practitioners, fully trained by the Bach Centre, who will help you to understand the "type" of person you are and to decide the most suitable remedy for you.

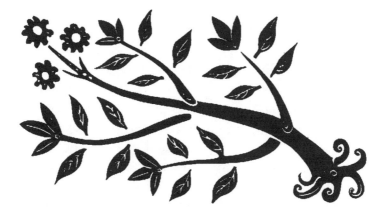

Perhaps the best-known Bach remedy is the rescue remedy, recommended in times of crisis and as an aid to the relief of shock and trauma caused by physical, emotional, or mental injury and illness. These may include accidents to oneself or to one's loved ones, animal and insect bites, burns, scalds, and pre- and postsurgery upset. A combination of cherry plum, clematis, impatiens, rock rose, and star of Bethlehem, it is available in liquid and cream form.

Other Bach remedies include: crab apple to ease, among other things, feelings of shame about ailments such as eczema; elm to overcome feelings of inadequacy; mimulus for those who are shy, nervous, or afraid; pine to counteract self-blame and feelings of guilt; scleranthus to overcome indecision and mood swings; and willow to counteract bitterness and feelings of self-pity.

The remedies can be bought from health-food stores and suppliers of natural medicine, or from the Bach Centre.

What they are used for

The remedies have been used to treat agoraphobia; anxiety; bites and stings; bruises; minor burns; claustrophobia; depression; fainting; fear; hysteria; mood swings; nervous disorders; panic attacks; phobias; premenstrual tension; postnatal depression; psychosomatic illnesses; sexual problems; stammering; stress; temper tantrums; and tension. They are also used to treat emotional aspects associated with acne, addictions, allergies, amnesia, asthma, bulimia, chronic fatigue syndrome, eczema, psoriasis, and other physical diseases in which emotional suffering is involved.

What doctors think

Scientists remain baffled by how these remedies work, as chemical analyses reveal only water and alcohol.

BEHAVIORAL THERAPY

Origins

Russian scientist Ivan Pavlov conditioned animals to behave in certain ways so that he could better understand human behavior, using techniques today known as *conditioning*. An American, J. B. Watson, worked along similar lines and called his theories *behaviorism*.

Another American, psychologist B. F. Skinner, expanded the theories, eventually proposing the process of *reinforcement:* the setting or solidifying of certain behavior patterns through experience of and expectation of certain results, such as rewards and punishments. Some of Skinner's ideas are still in use today to treat such disorders as claustrophobia. With this disorder, for example, instead of "allowing" the fear of confined spaces to be reinforced as a terrifying, unpleasant experience, it is reinforced as a pleasant, cozy, womblike, and secure experience.

The work of these scientists, and others, became the foundation for the field of behavioral therapy.

What it is

Every parent, teacher, and lover knows what behavioral therapy is—the encouraging of acceptable behavior through rewards, such as a smile, a hug, words of praise, and treats, and the discouraging of unacceptable behavior through frowns, finger wagging, words of correction, and punishments, such as loss of privileges. In other words, it is the changing of behavior through retraining.

In addition to psychotherapy, which is straightforwardly based on the above ideas, there are other forms of behavioral therapy.

Aversion Therapy

Aversion therapy is based on the principle of learning through self-punishment. The therapy uses a nausea-inducing drug, which causes a person to be horribly sick every time he or she gives in to a particular addiction, such as alcohol, drugs, or smoking. Success usually depends on the person's desire to give up the habit and to be cured of the addiction.

Encounter Group Therapy

See page 69

Flooding (Forced Exposure)

A short, sharp form of shock therapy, flooding works on the principle that dread and fear can be exhausted and de-fused. In this therapy, the person is continually exposed to his or her own particular fear until he or she no longer experiences terror. Ghastly though it sounds, many claims are made for its effectiveness in curing phobias, such as the fear of spiders and vertigo.

Imaging Aversion Therapy

Imaging aversion therapy works on the same principle as aversion therapy but is considered less extreme. Instead of taking a nausea-inducing drug, you imagine something extremely unpleasant in lieu of your particular addiction—like drinking urine instead of whisky, or putting a blood-drenched cigarette into your mouth. It is said help break antisocial and dangerous habits.

Systematic Desensitization

In systematic desensitization, the therapist encourages the person to dwell on his or her worst fear and then introduces relaxation techniques to counteract or overcome the fear. Gradually, through a process of tension and relaxation, tension and relaxation, desensitization occurs.

What it is used for

Behavioral therapy is used to help addiction; agoraphobia; anxiety; antisocial behavior (such as indecent exposure and shoplifting); children's bedwetting, school phobias, and truancy; claustrophobia; disruptive behaviors (such as hyperactivity); stress-induced headaches; insomnia; irrational fears; nervous disorders; obsessive and compulsive behavior; panic attacks;

phobias; psychosomatic illnesses; sexual problems; sleep disorders; smoking; stress; temper tantrums; tension; tics; and vertigo.

What doctors think

Many doctors believe that behavioral therapy reaches problems and disorders that orthodox treatments cannot reach, and are therefore in favor of it, especially of psychotherapists. Others express suspicion that more extreme forms, such forced exposure to fears, might tip the balance between borderline normalcy and serious mental illness.

BIOCHEMIC TISSUE SALTS THERAPY

Origins

This therapy was developed in the 1870s by a German homeopathic doctor, W. H. Schuessler. The terms *biochemic* and *tissue salts* were coined by Schuessler to help describe the effects of twelve tissue salts that he named in the body.

What it is

Biochemic tissue salts therapy is essentially a self-help treatment based on the widely researched fact that the cells need the right balance of natural mineral salts to stay healthy and that a lack or imbalance leads to common ailments. Maintaining the balance and restoring deficiencies is what this particular therapy is intended to do.

Apart from Schuessler's original list of twelve tissue salts (listed with a number, chemical name, and common name, such as *4 Ferr phos. Iron phosphate*, some biochemic tissue salts have been

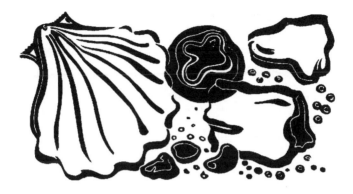

combined by practitioners to treat common ailments, such as menstrual pain and heartburn. These remedies are designated with a letter of the alphabet; for example, Combination B.

Herbalists, homeopaths, and naturopaths often prescribe biochemic tissue salts to complement other alternative therapies.

Biochemic tissue salts can be bought from pharmacies and health-food stores, and are mostly produced at the low potency of 6X. The tissue salts that you take will depend on the prevailing condition that either you or your therapist has noted.

What it is used for

Biochemic tissue salts therapy is used for a multitude of ailments and disorders, including acidity; acne; agoraphobia; anxiety; arthritis; asthma; bladder problems; blisters; boils; bronchitis; catarrh; chicken pox; circulation problems; colds; coughs; cramps; cystitis; digestive problems; fever; glandular fever; gout; hay fever; heartburn; indigestion; influenza; lumbago; manic-depressive illness; menstrual problems; migraines; mineral deficiency; mumps; muscular pain; nausea and vomiting; nerve disorders; neuralgia; neuritis; pain; panic attacks; pimples; prostate problems; sciatica; thrush; vaginitis; and wheezing.

What doctors think

Doctors express concern that treatment for serious illness should not be delayed by belief in this therapy. They also add that although it is medically accepted that at least twelve tissue salts are at work in the body and are essential to the maintenance of good health, this does not confirm that biochemic tissue salts can effectively treat all the ailments that the therapy claims to treat.

Warning

The tablets are lactose based; anyone suffering from milk-sugar allergies or lactose intolerance should take this into account.

BIOENERGETICS

Origins

Dr. Alexander Lowen, an American, was a pupil of the maverick Freudian psychoanalyst Dr. Wilhelm Reich, who was jailed by U.S. medical authorities for continuing to sell equipment and publish theories of which they disapproved. In the 1960s, Lowen drew on some aspects of Reich's work to develop his own theories of bioenergetics. His theories have since earned the approval and respect of many modern psychotherapists.

What it is

Bioenergetics is a way of understanding the personality in terms of the body and its energetic processes, including breathing, movement, feeling, sexuality, and self-expression.

Lowen developed active exercises for releasing chronically tense muscles. Some emphasize emotional expression, while others highlight deepening contact with the body, particularly the legs and pelvis. Much work is done in a standing position to increase grounding—the ability to stand on one's own two feet. A particularly well-known exercise is called the bow. In this exercise, one bends the knees and, while turning the toes inward, pushes the pelvis forward using the fists at the small of the back. In this position, vibrations created by a positive musculoskeletal stress start to build up the energetic charge of the body.

Bioenergetics is practiced in exercise classes, in therapy groups, and in individual sessions with a therapist.

What it is used for

Bioenergetics helps people free themselves from limitations and develop their full potential through increasing self-awareness.

Success is also claimed for helping people who suffer from asthma; headaches; migraines; psychosomatic problems; stress-related ailments and disorders; unresolved states of shock; and wheezing.

What doctors think

As bioenergy cannot be measured scientifically, many doctors remain skeptical.

BIOFEEDBACK THERAPY

Origins   The origins of biofeedback go back to the beginning of this century when, for example, psychologist Carl Jung used the measurement of galvanic skin resistance to monitor changes in the nervous system of his patients, which he associated with subconscious emotional responses. It became more popular with the advent of transistor and modern electronics, which opened the door to more sophisticated instruments for monitoring subtle changes in psychological states.

Most of the instruments used in this therapy were originally designed for use in medical and scientific research. Perhaps the most famous biofeedback instrument is, thanks to Hollywood, the lie detector that is so beloved of homicide and espionage investigations.

What it is   Biofeedback is a way of learning to be more aware of mental, emotional, and physical responses that are often beyond normal consciousness, but that can have a detrimental influence on health and well-being.

The biofeedback practitioner uses instruments to give you clear signals of your responses. These include measurement of muscle tension with an electromyograph (EMG), measurement of brain-wave patterns with an electroencephalograph (EEG), and measurement of nervous activity with a skin-resistance meter.

The underlying principle of biofeedback therapy is that changes in thinking and emotion will effect corresponding changes in the body.

Measuring physical changes gives the practitioner and you an objective view of their emotional and mental counterparts. For example, chronic tension in the neck and head can be monitored with an EMG, which measures the motor-neuron activity in these muscles. You can then discover how changing your thinking or attention can reduce this tension.

What it is used for

Biofeedback therapy is useful for any psychosomatic ailment including anxiety symptoms; asthma; breathing disorders (such as hyperventilation); high blood pressure; hypnotherapy; migraines; tension headaches; and as an aid to relaxation methods such as autogenics, breathing techniques, and meditation.

What doctors think

Biofeedback is finding its way into conventional medicine and is, for example, included in recommended treatments for heart disease. It is being introduced in simple forms by doctors and anti-stress and rehabilitation clinics.

BREATHING FOR RELAXATION THERAPY

Origins

As old as the first life on earth and part of many ancient healing practices, breathing for relaxation is supported by much current scientific research.

What it is

Breathing for relaxation therapy consists of a series of breathing exercises specifically designed to help a person to relax the body and mind.

The two primary breathing methods are chest breathing and diaphragmatic breathing. Ideally, chest breathing, which delivers a quick inhalation of oxygen, should be used only as an initial response to sudden tension, shock, or stress. Unfortunately, chest breathing often becomes the only form of breathing, resulting in the fast, shallow pants so obvious in people who are anxious, fearful, stressed, and hyperventilating (overbreathing). When chest breathing becomes habitual, the stress it creates takes its toll on general health, with a consequent breakdown of physical, emotional, and mental well-being.

Diaphragmatic breathing is natural, rhythmic breathing that allows a fuller expansion of the lungs and a decrease in the buildup of waste products, such as carbon dioxide and lactic acid, that can cause or exacerbate exhaustion and nervousness.

Breathing techniques are taught in standing, sitting, and reclining positions, and loose clothing is recommended. Once the basic breathing techniques have been mastered, they are typically practiced in fifteen-minute daily sessions in a quiet setting.

What it is used for

As with all other relaxation techniques, the purpose of correct breathing is to reduce the negative effects of excessive stress in body and mind. It is used to improve physical, emotional, and mental well-being, and is especially recommended for counteracting exhaustion, general nervousness, insomnia, respiratory disorders, shock, stress, trauma, and tiredness. People who work in high-pressure, stressful jobs can certainly benefit from learning such techniques.

What doctors think

Breathing deeply has always been considered the most effective way to counteract both short- and long-term tension and stress-related problems. The medical profession is generally aware that patients reveal much about themselves by the way they breathe—for example, quick, shallow breathing from the upper chest may indicate emotional and mental disturbance, as well as physical disorders.

BRISTOL DIET THERAPY

See Diet Therapies

CHILDBIRTH AND PREGNANCY

See Special Needs section, pages 214 to 217

CHIROPRACTIC

See also Osteopathy

Origins

David Daniel Palmer (1845–1913), a hands-on healer, founded the Palmer School of Chiropractic after proving to himself and others that manipulation of misaligned bones within the spine could correct a variety of disorders. Palmer described the painful conditions he treated as originating in "displacement of the skeletal frame," resulting in physical mobility problems, pressure on various nerves, muscle spasm, locked joints, tender joints, and pain.

What it is

Loosely translated, *chiropractic* means "practice by hand," and although it is similar to osteopathy, chiropractors rely more than osteopaths on orthodox diagnostic techniques such as X rays.

Chiropractors use their hands to manipulate the joints of the spine and to place slight pressure and rapid thrusts on vertebrae. This stretches muscles, unlocks joints, and corrects problems in other parts of the body that have originated from the spine. In addition to joint manipulation, a chiropractor sometimes applies heat, ice, or ultrasound to affected areas.

Treatment does not usually begin until the chiropractor has studied the spine, noted signs of injury or disease, and decided whether the person is a suitable candidate for chiropractic treatment and if an X ray is necessary. For the actual treatment, the person may be sitting, standing, or lying on a specially designed chiropractic couch. For some people, relief is immediate; others may need three or four treatments before relief is experienced. Some people experience general aches and soreness after the treatment.

Chiropractors sometimes discover injuries stemming from childhood falls and accidents or untreated whiplash injuries. The person may have made physical adjustments—changed the natural way of moving to neutralize untreated discomfort and pain—that may have resulted in misalignment of the spine and subsequent health problems.

What it is used for

Chiropractic is primarily employed for back pain, headaches, migraines, and bone and joint problems. Visceral conditions have been known to respond to manipulation carried out by a chiropractor.

What doctors think

Earlier negative attitudes have given way to positive responses concerning treatment of musculoskeletal problems, and doctors are increasingly referring patients to chiropractors. The Medical Research Council in Great Britain carried out a three-year trial comparing chiropractic treatment with conventional treatment for back pain and found chiropractic treatment 70 percent more effective.

COUNSELING

See also Psychotherapy

What it is   Counselors offer people the time, attention, and respect necessary to explore and clarify ways of living more resourcefully and with greater well-being. Emphasis is placed on confidentiality, respect for the client's own perception of his or her experience, and support for the client to find his or her own solutions to difficulties. Depending on a person's concern, a particular type of counselor may be appropriate. Counseling specializations include mental health, couples and family counseling, rehabilitation, and educational counseling. As with psychotherapy, different analytic methods may be used; however, counselors tend to adopt a "whatever works" approach rather than following a particular therapeutic method.

What it is used for   Counseling therapy is commonly recommended for people who have experienced shock and trauma as a result of being involved in, or close to someone who has been involved in, a traumatic disaster, such as an earthquake or a car or airplane accident. It is also recommended for victims of crime and other forms of violence.

Counseling is also used to treat anxiety, depression, mood swings, and other personal issues that would benefit from detached guidance. Counselors take pains to explain that "detached" never means "cold indifference." It means somebody who is trained to listen without becoming so emotionally involved that the counseling is ineffective.

The choice of a counselor will depend on whether you simply want a "listening ear" for a general problem, or a person who specializes, for example, in counseling victims of rape, people who have family problems (such as a compulsive gambler or drug addict within the family), or people with suicidal tendencies.

What doctors think

Only too conscious that they lack the time necessary to deal in depth with emotional and mental problems, doctors are very positive about the value of counseling and psychotherapy, and frequently recommend them to their patients.

CRANIOSACRAL THERAPY

Origins

The founder of cranial osteopathy, Dr. William Garner Sutherland, saw life as movement and pulsation, expansion and contraction; he called these movements "the breath of life." Sutherland developed manipulation techniques for the skull and facial bones to allow "the breath of life" to express itself more fully in the body and to reestablish its presence wherever it had been impeded.

What it is

Craniosacral therapy is a deeply relaxing healing system in which the practitioner, through gentle procedures of touch, listens to the body's movements, rhythms, pulsations, and patterns of congestion and resistance. The therapy assists the body's natural healing processes and increases vitality and well-being. Patients may become aware of alterations in fluid pressures, tissue release, heat, tingling, and energy releases.

Many treatments take place with the patient lying down, although some procedures use sitting or standing positions to unravel tensions and resistance in the joints and connective tissues.

Practitioners believe that the whole of our life history is held in our physical form. They believe that a current disease process or pain may have its roots in very early experience, such as birth trauma, when compressive forces can cause imbalances in the craniosacral system.

What it is used for

This gentle therapy, which is suitable for babies, children, and adults, including the elderly, is used to treat very fragile or acutely painful conditions.

What doctors think

The general feeling of doctors toward craniosacral therapy is positive when the treatment is practiced by a qualified osteopath who, before starting manipulation, establishes that the symptoms are not caused by infection, a fracture, or a tumor.

CYMATIC THERAPY

See also Sound Therapy

Origins

Dr. Peter Manners originated this therapy in the 1960s.

What it is	Cymatic therapy is a sound-wave therapy that stimulates areas of the body through the use of a handheld applicator, pads, or plates that aim high-frequency sounds to specific parts of the body for healing purposes. Treatment may also include sound waves transmitted into a water pool warmed to body temperature.
What it is used for	Cymatic therapy is used for arthritis; bone fractures; gout; lumbago; postsurgery healing; rheumatism; sciatica; slipped disc; sports injuries; and stress-related tension.
What doctors think	Cymatic therapy is now used in some orthopedic hospitals to assist in the treatment of such things as bone fractures.

DANCE MOVEMENT THERAPY

Origins	In the 1940s, when dancers and movement specialists such as Rudolph Laban and Marian Chase began to use dance movements to help people with emotional problems, the idea of dance as a therapy began to attract attention, particularly in the United States and Europe.
What it is	The therapy is a form of communication that is not dependent on words, a body language expressed through dance movements. The person does not need to be able to dance or to have any previous dance experience. The sessions always begin with movements everybody can manage and enjoy. The warm-up period allows muscles to

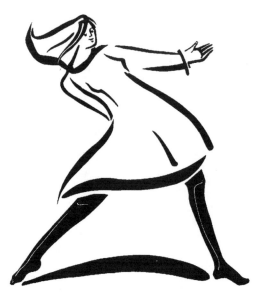

relax. It is followed by movements suggested by the therapist, and then people are encouraged to innovate their own movements, with or without the accompaniment of music.

Throughout each session the therapist is on hand to encourage and help individuals to find new ways to express themselves and, if the individual wishes and is able, to discuss the emotions—anger, anguish, fear, grief, jealousy, laughter, love—that "direct" any particular sequence of movements.

As confidence increases, individuals can continue to explore and, with gentle encouragement, make discoveries about themselves through the movements. Inhibitions and repressions may be shed, and new abilities to relate and come closer to others may be discovered.

What it is
used for
Dance therapy is particularly recommended for children with physical disabilities (for example, blindness, deafness, or muteness); children with learning problems, sometimes resulting in behavioral problems (for example, aggressive and disruptive behavior, hyperactivity, or an inability to concentrate); adolescents struggling with pent-up emotions or neuroses (such as anorexia and bulimia); people who have communication problems; people who have difficulties forming relationships; and people who are mentally ill.

What doctors
think
Many doctors agree that dance therapy is emotionally and psychologically helpful for people with physical and mental disabilities or who are mentally ill, and for children and adults with behavioral and communication problems. As yet it is not a regulated profession.

DIET THERAPIES

Diet therapies are intended to address specific health concerns and to generally support good health through a planned course of food and nutrition.

BRISTOL DIET

Origins
The Bristol diet was devised by Dr. Alex Forbes as a strict vegan, raw-food diet. Named after the Bristol Cancer Self-Help Centre where it was first used, the diet has been modified to include more

cooked food, and some fish, free-range chicken, eggs, and organically farmed meat. Great emphasis is placed on fresh vegetables and fruit, whole grains and legumes (beans, lentils, and peas), and organically produced goat's yogurt.

Herb teas, freshly pressed juices, and spring water are recommended instead of tea and coffee. Herbs and spices replace salt and pepper. Cold-pressed or virgin olive oil is used for cooking.

What it is used for   The clinic uses the Bristol diet, in addition to counseling, meditation, and other therapies, to help cancer patients enhance their quality of life.

GERSON THERAPY DIET

Origins   Max Gerson, a 1920s German physician, devised this therapy to treat his migraine. He was so impressed he recommended it to his patients, and even people with tuberculosis and cancer have claimed that it helped.

What it is   The diet therapy is based on drinking glasses of freshly pressed vegetable and fruit juices (primarily carrot juice) every hour. Caffeine enemas and castor oil are recommended to help cleanse the body; food, which must be organically grown, is primarily salad, oats, and baked potatoes in their skins.

The diet is intended to eliminate the buildup of toxins in the body by stimulating enzymes, improving the digestive system, and ensuring the right balance of vitamins and minerals. The diet is said to promote a positive attitude to oneself and to life.

What doctors think   Doctors generally regard this as an extreme diet and believe there are ways of finding relief without such unpleasant side effects.

Warning   The therapy usually causes nausea and diarrhea and, while this is considered part of the cleansing process, such symptoms can be exceedingly unpleasant.

HAY DIET THERAPY

Origins   Ivan Pavlov, a Russian physiologist, discovered that meat eaten with starchy foods take twice as long to pass through an animal's stomach as meat or carbohydrate eaten alone. It was from this research that the American doctor William Howard devised the Hay diet.

What it is   The Hay diet maintains that carbohydrates—starchy and sweet foodstuffs—should be eaten at separate mealtimes from proteins and acidic fruits. The diet also recommends that carbohydrates and proteins not be eaten within four hours of each other. Pulses (beans, lentils, and peas) and peanuts are excluded from the diet.

For acidic fruit, Howard suggested fresh and dried apples, apricots, gooseberries, oranges, pears, and prunes. For carbohydrates, he listed whole-grain bread, flour, rice, bananas, dried fruits (dates, figs, currants, raisins, sultanas) and, for vegetables, potatoes and Jerusalem artichokes. For protein, he included cheese, fish, eggs, meat, milk, poultry, shellfish, and yogurt.

For his neutral food group—that is, food that can be eaten with any of the other groups—he included butter, cream, egg yolks, nuts (except for peanuts), oil (olive, safflower, and sesame), salads, seeds (sunflower and sesame), vegetables (green and root, except for potatoes and Jerusalem artichokes).

In addition to eating acidic fruits, carbohydrates, and protein separately, refined and processed foods (such as sugar and white flour), are banned, and great emphasis is placed on increasing fruit, salad, and vegetables in the diet and reducing carbohydrates, fats, and proteins.

You are allowed, in moderation, beer, gin, or whisky with carbohydrate meals, and wine, cider, gin, or whisky with protein meals.

What it is used for

The Hay diet is intended to encourage good all-around health and well-being and to prevent the problems of obesity, including high blood pressure and heart disease; arthritis; constipation; diabetes; indigestion; ulcers (stomach and duodenal).

What doctors think

This diet is less extreme and sounds better balanced than many of the diets doctors' patients mention. Few, however, support the idea of separating foods by class.

HEALTHY LIVING DIET THERAPY

Origins   Hippocrates, the father of modern medicine, is quoted as saying: "Let food be your medicine and medicine be your food." Ancient Chinese physicians began healing by considering a patient's diet. The World Health Organization presses home the virtues of a healthful diet and its contribution to counteracting a host of modern-day diseases.

There is endless publicity in magazines and newspapers repeating what everyone already knows: that "we are what we eat," that an inadequate diet leads to poor health and that a healthful diet leads to good health, a general sense of well-being, a positive attitude, and a much better chance of achieving one's potential, physically, mentally, and emotionally.

What it is Most healthy living diets have the following in common: They are usually vegetarian, or recommend a high proportion of fresh vegetables and fruit in relation to fish and meat. They place

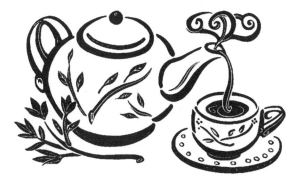

great emphasis on organically grown vegetables and fruit, and whole-grain products, such as bread, oats, pasta, and rice. Raw food is often considered preferable to cooked, and a high proportion of raw food is recommended. A reduction in the use of sugar, salt and pepper, and caffeine is recommended.

What it is used for

There is much research and other evidence that bowel, breast, and stomach cancers are less common in societies where the diet is high in fiber (for example, vegetables, fruits, and whole-grain cereals), which aid the swift elimination of waste products, and low in fat and meat, which tend to have harmful, sluggish effects on the body's systems. Swift elimination of waste products is considered so important because cancer-causing substances are hurried through and out of the system before they have the chance to create health problems.

MACROBIOTIC DIET THERAPY

Origins

The idea behind the macrobiotic diet is that eating a diet that promotes physical, mental, emotional, and spiritual health and harmony will encourage us to live life to our full potential. Its origins lie in the work of a Japanese doctor, Sagen Ishizuka, who believed in treating a variety of health problems with what later became known as "organic health foods"—whole-grain cereals and vegetables. Another Japanese, George Ohsawa, who was convinced that his tuberculosis was cured by Ishizuka's diet, carried the work forward by writing a book on what he called macrobiotics. The word *macrobiotic* is based on the Greek word derived from using *macros*, meaning long, and *bios*, meaning life, which was first used by Hippocrates.

What it is

Drawing on the Chinese philosophy of yin and yang, the macrobiotic diet aims to balance foods for their yin-yang qualities and to balance the food to the yin-yang qualities of the individual. The primary goal is to eat foods in the middle range—such as grains, which are neither extreme yin nor yang—and thereby achieve a healthy and harmonious life.

A macrobiotic food cupboard would include the following, preferably organically grown: whole-grain cereals (including barley, bread, buckwheat, corn, couscous, millet, oats, pasta, rice, and wheat); fruit (fresh, preferably in season, and dried); oils (polyunsaturated and monounsaturated—sunflower oil and virgin olive oil are great favorites); juices (pure, savory, and sweet, but minus additives and sweeteners); nuts; pulses (beans, peas, lentils); seeds (sunflower seeds are popular); herbal tisanes; vegetables (freshly grown and picked, and eaten in their appropriate season); and spring water.

Many vegetarians use macrobiotic diets, but other people include fresh seafood and fish in their macrobiotic diet.

As much emphasis is placed on cooking utensils as on the food itself. Cast-iron pots and pans are preferred because they distribute heat more evenly. Steamer sets are recommended for cooking vegetables because little water is needed, and what water is left can be used in soups and sauces, so the process is more efficient at retaining nutrients.

What it is used for

Success, backed up by case histories, has been claimed for treating and curing arthritis, digestive problems, and cancer. Although it is claimed that the diet will help in the prevention and treatment of most common ailments and diseases, it is also recommended for the healthy and for warding off illness.

What doctors think

Do not be surprised if your doctor is against the macrobiotic diet. Many family doctors remember the publicity the diet attracted in the 1960s and 1970s, when some people took it to a dangerous extreme for themselves and their children and ate nothing but brown rice.

Warning

Pregnant women, people in poor health, mothers who are breastfeeding, and parents who are considering placing children on macrobiotic diets are advised to consult their family doctors first.

NUTRITIONAL THERAPY

Origins

In the late nineteenth century and early twentieth century, naturopaths began to use nutrition and fasting, together with other therapies, to cleanse the body and to help build up its self-healing ability. By the 1950s much

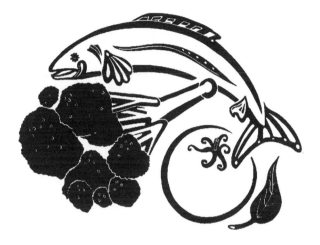

more knowledge had been gained about the composition of food, and specialist practitioners of nutritional therapy (at first mainly doctors) began to devise diets and regimes of vitamins and minerals for specific symptoms and illnesses.

What it is   Nutritional therapy is a sophisticated health-care system that uses a knowledge of physiology and body chemistry to achieve a desired therapeutic effect by directing a patient's nutrition. The therapist works on a basis of three broad diagnoses: allergies, toxic overload, and nutritional deficiencies.

Diagnosis is made through questioning and examining the patient, after which the patient is given a treatment regime. The prescribed diet will vary according to individual needs, and supplements may be included as well as basic herbs and herbal teas. The initial, sometimes restrictive diet may last for ten weeks, although the full healing process may take several months.

What it is used for

Practitioners believe that every part of the body is made from what was once food. The aim is to explore how an individual's health has gone wrong and to help that person understand how to correct it through nutrition. Nutritional therapy can play an important part in developing the body's strength and resistance.

What doctors think

Interest and support for nutritional therapy is steadily growing, worldwide.

RAW FOOD DIET THERAPY

Origins

Long known as the "nature cure" diet beloved of naturopaths, the raw food diet is now entering its second century of popular use. However, if one considers that human beings must have eaten before the discovery of fire and the means to cook, the raw food diet could be considered as old as the human race itself.

What it is

The raw food diet consists of raw fruit and vegetables, eaten fresh and in season, and supplemented with muesli (uncooked cereal), nuts, pulses (beans, peas, and lentils), seeds (pumpkin and sunflower), and sprouting grains.

Naturopaths believe that a diet that relies heavily on meat undermines the human digestive tract's ability to cope and that, as a result, food takes too long to pass through the body, releasing harmful toxins into the system. They also believe that vital, health-enhancing enzymes, fiber, minerals, nutrients, and vitamins are lost in the cooking process; that fruits and vegetables are alkali forming and desirable for good health; and that dairy products, egg yolks, fish, and meat are acid forming and undesirable for good health.

What doctors think

Most doctors appreciate a raw diet's therapeutic value but prefer, especially where children are concerned, the inclusion of dairy products, cooked pulses, oily fish, and some meat to ensure the widest possible range of nutrients.

VEGANISM

What it is

Frequently confused with vegetarianism, veganism has one crucial fundamental difference; it is a vegetables-and-fruit-only diet. Vegans do not eat *any* animal products such as butter, cheese, or eggs.

What doctors think

As a whole, doctors are much more at ease with a vegetarian diet than a vegan diet, and will certainly talk about the need for protein and the value of dairy products, especially if children are being raised as vegans.

Warning

Vegans can be deficient in calcium, iron, zinc, and vitamin B12. Severe depletion of vitamin B12 may result in nerve disorders, brain damage, or anemia. Many vegans use yeast-extract products or take supplements to counteract the lack of vitamins and minerals in their diet.

Breastfeeding mothers on a vegan diet should consult their doctor, as their baby may need a vitamin B12 supplement.

VEGETARIANISM

What it is   A vegetarian diet, as the name implies, is mainly vegetable in origin but includes quantities of whole-grain cereals, pulses (beans, peas, and lentils), and fresh and dried fruit and nuts. Unlike vegans, with whom they are often confused, vegetarians also eat animal products, such as butter, cheese, eggs, and milk. Their diet is considered less extreme than a vegan diet, which can be lacking in calcium, iron, zinc, and vitamin B12.

People who do not eat meat but who include fish in their diet are often referred to as "partial" vegetarians. The term is also applied to people who do not eat any red meat but who occasionally eat chicken.

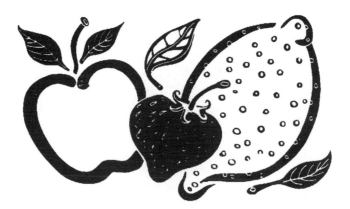

A varied diet is vital if vegetarians are to ensure they are receiving their full quota of nutrients. Preparing a kitchen chart that displays sources for the essential nutrients—calcium, protein, iron, zinc, vitamin B12, and vitamin C—is an excellent idea. These are frequently published in health magazines and newspaper health supplements, and information can be obtained from the relevant organizations. The following balanced dietary approach is typical: four daily helpings of carbohydrates (such as bread, cereals, pasta, potatoes, and rice); fruit and vegetables; and protein (such as cheese, eggs, pulses, and nuts).

What it is used for

Vegetarianism is often associated with a low incidence of blood pressure problems and there is a growing belief that a well-balanced, meatless diet is good for promoting health and well-being.

What doctors think

Few doctors criticize vegetarianism as a health hazard, and many agree that, provided it is balanced to include all the nutrients for healthy growth and maintenance, it has many advantages.

Warning

Vegetarian women who suffer from menstrual problems, such as bleeding between periods or heavy blood loss during menstruation, should seek medical advice about a possible iron-deficiency problem.

ELECTROTHERAPY

See also Galvanism

Origins

Electrotherapy is thought to have been inspired by a doctor in ancient Rome, who treated a patient's inflamed and swollen foot by placing it on a live electric eel. Later, nineteenth-century doctors took to relieving an assortment of aches and pains by discharging an electric current through the appropriate part of the body. Dentists subsequently used a pain-reducing electric current when extracting teeth. The procedure has been refined and is in general use in Japan.

What it is

In one kind of electrotherapy, known as TNS (transcutaneous nerve stimulation), nerves are stimulated to block out pain. The patient has jelly-coated rubber pads attached to the appropriate area of the body, and a gentle electrical current is passed through the pads into the skin.

There is also a form of acupuncture in which the TNS machine is used to pass electrical pulses through needle pressure points.

What it is used for

Today the therapy is often used by hospital physiotherapists, in maternity hospitals, and by physiotherapists in private practice to assist with childbirth; circulation problems; lumbago; sciatica; weight loss; sports injuries; stress incontinence that sometimes follows childbirth; and surgical procedures.

A handheld machine, described as an electrical stimulator, can be bought for self-help procedures, but it is not considered as successful as the TNS machines used by the medical profession and complementary treatment practitioners.

What doctors think
Doctors value electrotherapy as a pain-relieving treatment, but ewe are convinced of its value as a weight-loss aid. Many have serious doubts about the effectiveness of a self-help electrical stimulator.

Warning
TNS machines interfere with the workings of heart pacemakers, so people who have these should not use this therapy.

Before embarking on a course of electric acupuncture, you are advised to consult your family doctor.

ENCOUNTER GROUP THERAPY

See also Behavioral Therapy

Origins
Carl Rogers, an American psychologist, was the main instigator of encounter group therapy. Having spent years in one-to-one encounters, he became convinced around the 1940s that group encounters could free more people more quickly and that group interaction could reveal underlying personality problems and promote resolutions.

Today the therapy has expanded from its once exclusive use in psychiatric establishments to use by nonmedically qualified people. It is used in companies to encourage employees to interact better with each other and their business contacts and, having increased their self-understanding and awareness of other's needs, to fulfill their potential.

What it is
A "this above all to thine own self be true" therapy, the emphasis of encounter group therapy is on getting to know yourself and others better. This is done by understanding "undercurrents," the tug and tow of emotions such as resentment, suspicion, and anger that influence you and others.

Groups usually meet for several sessions a week or for an intensive one- or two-day session. Various means are used to relax the participants, to help them get to know each other, to build a sense of trust and to help them be as honest as possible about themselves and their feelings. The aim of encounter group therapy is to find positive resolutions to conflict and to rechannel

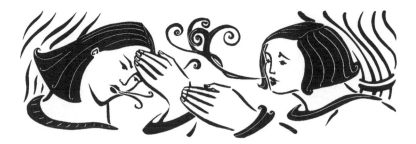

negative feelings into more beneficial, constructive, and fulfilling behavior.

Encounter groups, also called sensitivity groups, work successfully only when the constant challenging of individuals and their behavior and feelings is supported by the group.

What it is used for

Encounter groups are typically held for people who are already receiving medical treatment for emotional or mental disorders; people who are experiencing serious discord in personal relationships, perhaps as a result of divorce or domestic violence; and for people in business relationships.

What doctors think

If encounter groups are not conducted by qualified psychotherapists and if adequate ongoing support is not provided, doctors believe that more harm than good is likely to result, especially for emotionally vulnerable people.

EXERCISE THERAPIES

Specific exercise plans are used to treat a variety of conditions. Listed here are resources for several conditions known to benefit from exercise therapy.

Back Pain

Seek advice for relief of back pain from practitioners of acupressure, acupuncture, the Alexander technique, chiropractic, hypnotherapy, kinesiology, massage, osteopathy, physiotherapy, reflexology, Ta'i Chi Ch'uan, and yoga.

Balancing the Body's Energy Flow

For exercises intended to balance the flow of energy in the body, seek advice from practitioners of polarity therapy, T'ai Chi Ch'uan, and yoga.

Harmony of Body and Mind

Seek advice from practitioners of acupuncture, T'ai Chi Ch'uan, yoga, and Zen about exercises to increase the harmony between body and mind.

Neck Pain

To relieve neck pain, seek advice from practitioners of acupuncture, the Alexander technique, chiropractic, kinesiology, massage, osteopathy, physiotherapy, reflexology, and yoga.

Pregnancy

Breathing and relaxation exercises, physiotherapy, and yoga are used to relieve pain and tension associated with pregnancy, but ask your doctor's advice before commencing any exercise program.

Postnatal Period

Breathing and relaxation exercises, physiotherapy, yoga, and T'ai Chi Ch'uan are

used during the postnatal period, but ask your
doctor's advice before starting.

FASTING

Origins   Documented in the Bible and recommended by
ancient Greeks such as Socrates, Plato, and
Herodotus, fasting has been practiced throughout
time. Besides its use as a physical health remedy,
it has been used in many religions for spiritual
purposes to purify the mind as well as the body.

What it is   Fasting is a voluntary abstinence from eating. It
gives the digestive system a rest and allows the
body to rid itself of toxins and metabolic wastes.
Some believe the immune system is strengthened
as the body cleans out chemical toxins and dead
and damaged cells. Fasting also helps us to
understand the role food plays in our lives.
When eating is removed from our daily schedule,
we may find that we often eat to relieve stress or
boredom rather than for nourishment and relief
from hunger.

One approach to fasting is a partial fast,
which allows juices, while strict fasts only allow
water. The argument for partial fasts is that juices
provide vitamins and minerals yet are easily
digestible, which makes a fast less strenuous. A
fast commonly lasts one to three days, although
the body can survive for longer periods of time
as long as plenty of water is consumed. The
duration of a longer fast will depend on your
energy reserves and the activity levels you sustain

during the fast. Longer fasts should be discussed with a health professional. Depending on the length of a fast, medications you are taking may need to be adjusted or may prohibit fasting. Fasting should never be used for weight loss.

General guidelines include resting to allow the body to concentrate on the task of eliminating wastes, drinking 4 to 8 pints of water to flush out the system and reduce hunger pangs, and easing in and out of a fast, which helps the body adjust to the removal and reintroduction of food.

Some vitamin and mineral loss will occur during a fast, but a fairly healthy person will replenish these upon resuming a healthful diet.

What it is used for

In general, fasting is beneficial, especially for allergies, arthritis, constipation, headaches, heart disease, hypertension, inflammatory diseases, and psychological problems.

Warning

There are conditions for which fasting is not recommended, including diabetes, eating disorders, epilepsy, hypochondria, kidney disease, malnutrition, pregnancy, lactation, severe

bronchial asthma, terminal illness, tuberculosis, and ulcerative colitis.

FAMILY PLANNING THERAPY

See Special Needs section, page 211

FELDENKRAIS METHOD

Origins

The Israeli nuclear physicist Moshe Feldenkrais designed this therapy based on the idea that we each move, think, and feel in a different way and that the way we do each is in accord with the self-image that we have constructed over the years. Feldenkrais believed that we must change our self-image if we want to change our mode of action. If poor, habitual patterns of movement are overcome, the body will function more easily, which, in turn, will improve self- image, which will then increase awareness and health.

What it is

The Feldenkrais method is a two-stage therapy. The first stage is a hands-on session in which the practitioner uses touch to improve a person's breathing and body alignment. There is no attempt to structurally alter the body; instead, the practitioner shows the patient a different means by which the body can function through movement. This stage is formally called *functional integration.*

Secondly, through a series of floorwork classes of slow, nonaerobic movements, patients are taught correct ways to move their bodies to maintain the improvements from the hands-on work. The floorwork helps to integrate the mind and body. This stage is known as *awareness through movement.*

What it is used for
The Feldenkrais method is used to help alleviate the effects of stress, accidents, back problems, and physical diseases.

FLOWER ESSENCES THERAPIES

See Aromatherapy, Bach Flower Remedies

FLOTATION THERAPY

Origins
Flotation therapy stems from the ideas and experiments of American doctor, psychoanalyst, and neurophysiologist John Lilly, who was fascinated by what would happen if the human brain was cut off from all stimulation received through the five senses of hearing, sight, taste, touch, and smell. Working with an obliging colleague, Dr. Jay Shurley, Lilly experimented with floating the body in a tank of water removed from all other stimuli. In the 1970s, Lilly and Shurley pioneered the first flotation tank, similar to those used today, and publicized their theories.

What it is
The person being treated floats in an enclosed tank—sometimes called an isolation tank—of salt

and mineral water, in total or semidarkness. The theory is that when the brain is cut off from outside sensations and stimulation, a person is freed to become aware of his or her "inner" state of mind and being and to seek appropriate treatment or make appropriate adjustments to his or her lifestyle.

Practitioners of flotation therapy are often qualified in other therapies, such as counseling, meditation, and hypnotherapy.

Some flotation tanks are just for floating in, others are fitted with speakers to enable people to receive other forms of therapy while they float, and some include health-enhancing videos.

What it is used for

Flotation therapy is used to induce a state of self-awareness and total relaxation that increases understanding of what is needed to deal with such things as addiction, alcoholism, anxiety, insomnia, pain, tension, smoking, and relief from stress-related problems.

What doctors think

Flotation therapy should be used only under the careful supervision of an experienced practitioner.

Warning

Doctors consider this a dangerous therapy for people who are suffering from psychological disorders, such as manic depression and phobias. Consult your doctor if you are receiving treatment for emotional or psychological disturbances and stress-related ailments before trying flotation therapy.

GALVANISM

See also Electrotherapy

Origins

Galvanism was named after Luigi Galvani, an eighteenth-century anatomist who first spotted the medical potential in an electric current.

What it is

This electrotherapy treatment, which passes a direct current through electrodes rather than an alternating current through jelly-coated rubber pads, has been replaced by electrotherapy. It is included here because you may hear it referred to in complementary therapy circles.

GERSON THERAPY DIET

See Diet Therapies

GESTALT THERAPY

Origins   Gestalt counseling and therapy began in the early 1940s as a development of, and reaction to, psychoanalysis. It was cofounded by Fritz Perls (a Freudian psychoanalyst), Laura Perls (a psychologist), and Paul Goodman (a social philosopher and creative writer).

What it is   Gestalt is a holistic, relational, and versatile approach to counseling and psychotherapy. Its aim is to heighten people's perception of their current functioning in relation to other people and their environment, including behavior patterns of which they may not be aware. The Gestalt view is that people define, develop, and learn about their ever-changing selves in relationship to others. Sessions between therapist and client are intended to enable clients to share, develop, or change different aspects of themselves.

The Gestalt counselor designs imaginative and simple "experiments" in which the person tries out new behaviors and observes what happens. These may include creative elements such as silence, fantasy, visualization, role-playing, movement, drawing, and voice and language changes. Such experiments allow people to investigate their own behavior and increase their awareness of themselves and their surroundings.

What doctors think

When Gestalt therapy is performed by qualified practitioners, there is general consent among doctors that it can have beneficial and positive effects for individuals and their relationships with others.

HAY DIET THERAPY

See Diet Therapies

HEALTHY LIVING DIET THERAPY

See Diet Therapies

HELLERWORK THERAPY

Origins

Joseph Heller, an American aerospace engineer with an interest in structure, tension, and rigidity, applied his knowledge of aerodynamics to the human body and devised the Hellerwork therapy for realigning physical balance and improving body and mind integration.

What it is

The therapy has three components: bodywork (manipulation by the hands to release tension); dialogue (discussion on how habitual ideas, emotions, and strongly held views can influence physical, mental, and emotional factors); and movement education (counseling, plus guidance on increasing awareness of the body and how it is used, and on how to release the buildup of stresses and tensions).

The sessions are intensive, usually lasting about ninety minutes. In addition to the goals mentioned above, Hellerwork therapy works to free people from habitual rigid and health-threatening posture by realigning the natural balance on the fascia, a connective muscle-to-tendon-to-bone tissue.

What it is used for

Like the Alexander technique (see page 16), Hellerwork is a mind-body balance therapy, used primarily to prevent rather than to cure. As with the Alexander technique, people claim Hellerwork eases existing ailments and disorders.

What doctors think

Generally appreciative of the importance of good posture and movement, doctors find little to concern them here.

HERBAL MEDICINE

Origins

The origins of herbal medicine are as old as humans themselves. Its use can be traced back to Neanderthal society, ancient Egyptian priests, and the ancient Greeks and Romans, Chinese, and Indians. Until the eighteenth century it was the main form of medical treatment in the world.

What it is

As its name suggests, herbal medicine concerns the healing properties of medicinal herbs and plant-based medicines. Herbal medicines are extracted from flowers, fruit, leaves, roots, stems, and seeds.

Like naturopathy, herbalism places great emphasis on the holistic approach—treating every patient as an individual with distinct physical, emotional, medical, and spiritual needs—and concentrating on prevention as well as cure.

As people become increasingly aware of the dangerous side effects of some orthodox drug treatments, herbalism continues to increase in popularity.

What it is used for

Considered suitable for most common ailments and illnesses, success is claimed for treating acid stomach; acne; addiction; adenoids; agoraphobia; alcoholism; anemia; anal problems; anxiety; arteries (hardening of the); arthritis; asthma; athlete's foot; bad breath; bedwetting; bee stings; bladder problems; blisters; blood pressure (low and high); boils; bone fractures; bronchitis; bruising; bunions; bursitis; catarrh; celiac disease;

chicken pox; chronic fatigue syndrome; circulation problems; colds; colic; colitis; conjunctivitis; constipation; corns; coughs; cramps; croup; cystitis; dandruff; depression; diarrhea; earache; eczema; emphysema; exhaustion; eyestrain; fever; flatulence; fluid retention; food poisoning; frozen shoulder; fungal infections; gallstones; glandular fever; hangover; headaches; heat rash; hemorrhoids; hiccups; hives; impetigo; incontinence; indigestion; influenza; insomnia; irritable bowel syndrome; itching; jaundice; jet lag; laryngitis; measles; menopausal problems; menstrual problems; migraines; mood swings; morning sickness; mosquito bites; mumps; nausea and vomiting; nervous disorders; pain; panic attacks; phobias; pimples; premenstrual tension; prostate problems; psoriasis; rheumatism; ringing in the ears; sinus problems; sleep disorders; sneezing; stress; styes; sunburn; teeth grinding; temper tantrums; throat problems; thrush; thyroid problems; tonsillitis; tooth and gum disorders; ulcers (mouth, peptic, and varicose); vaginal disorders; viral infection; wasp stings; water retention; wheezing; whooping cough; and worms.

What doctors think

On the whole, doctors are appreciative of herbal medicine's contribution to treating common ailments, but less accepting when it comes to serious conditions. Now that so many modern drugs have serious side effects, the medical profession's attitude is generally less aggressive and negative, and many family doctors recommend herbal remedies.

HOMEOPATHY

Origins

Samuel Hahnemann, a brilliant German physician, made a name for himself in the worlds of medicine and science through his cooperation with other members of the medical profession and his work with chemists. His medical practice and research led him to question contemporary theories and practice; he had grave doubts about the efficacy of many treatments. When he discovered that he was sensitive to quinine and not allergic to it, he began to develop the theory of "like will be cured with like," which came to be the slogan of the homeopath.

What it is

Homeopathy is a holistic—involving body, mind, emotions, and spirit—approach that uses tiny doses of diluted substances to counteract health-threatening imbalances. The homeopathic doctor studies the whole person and takes into account idiosyncrasies; reactions to heat and cold, weather, and food; sleep and work patterns; age; and environment. The prime concern is the patient, not the symptoms. It is through this study and understanding of the way an individual's body reacts that allows remedies to be prescribed and healing to take place.

The remedies, which can be used by anyone, are available in powder, tincture, and tablet form in low- and high-potency doses. The success of homeopathy, however, requires a thorough knowledge of the remedy and the significance of the symptoms. Treatment by a homeopath who is thoroughly trained in medical diagnosis and pathology is essential.

Those sympathetic to homeopathy believe that the patient derives the greatest benefit when the principles of homeopathy are understood; a homeopath cannot help someone who continues to neglect or abuse his or her body.

What it is used for

Homeopathic remedies are used for acid stomach; acne; addiction; agoraphobia; allergies; anemia; anxiety; arthritis; asthma; bad breath; baldness; bee stings; bites (animal); bladder problems; blisters; blood pressure (high); boils; bronchitis; bruising; burns; bursitis; catarrh; chicken pox; chilblains; chronic fatigue syndrome; claustrophobia; cold sores; colds; colitis; conjunctivitis; constipation; coughs; cramps; cystitis; depression; diarrhea; earaches; eczema; exhaustion; eyestrain; fainting; fever; flatulence; food poisoning; frozen shoulder; fungal infections; gallstones; glandular fever; gout; grief; hangover; hay fever; headaches; heart disorders; hives; hyperactivity; influenza;

insomnia; irritable bowel syndrome; jaundice; kidney complaints; laryngitis; manic-depressive illness; measles; menopausal problems; menstrual problems; migraines; mood swings; mumps; nausea and vomiting; nervous disorders; obesity; panic attacks; phobias; piles; premenstrual tension; psoriasis; rheumatism; ringing in the ear; scalds; shingles; shock; sinus problems; sleep disorders; sports injuries; stress; sweating; throat problems; thyroid disorders; tiredness; tonsillitis; tooth and gum disorders; travel sickness; ulcers (leg, mouth, and peptic); vaginal disorders; viral infections; wheezing; and whooping cough.

What doctors think   Conflicts occur between traditional physicians and homeopaths because orthodox medicine relies on specific remedies for particular diseases, while homeopathy uses a variety of remedies to treat the whole person.

HUMANISTIC PSYCHOLOGY THERAPY

Origins   Carl Rogers and Abraham Maslow, two American psychologists, were the chief pioneers of humanistic psychology. Later, Carl Rogers devised Rogerian therapy (see page 128), which is strongly related to humanistic psychology.

Maslow was particularly interested in self-fulfillment—what it is that allows a person to be in harmony with himself or herself and to live life on the path of personal growth and fulfillment.

What it is   Humanistic psychology is based on the principle
                        that the belief in oneself, in one's potential for
                        lifelong personal growth and development, and
                        in one's personal problem-solving abilities is
                        essential for a fulfilling life experience.

What it is   Humanistic psychology seeks to help people
used for   achieve the above by concentrating the person
                        and the practitioner's energies on the current
                        problem and how the individual can tap positive
                        attitudes to free negative beliefs, effects, and
                        influences.

                        All types of humanistic psychology take the
                        view that, while we are subject to many
                        influences—genetic, family, environmental, and
                        social—we are not the helpless products of
                        negative forces. We have within us the strength to
                        resolve negation and to take charge of our own
                        life and development. For this reason, humanistic
                        psychologists do not go in for deep
                        psychoanalysis of babyhood, childhood, and past
                        experiences, but concentrate their healing
                        approach and the person's energies on the
                        immediate issue. Your fulfillment is in your
                        hands and not at the mercy of divine or human
                        forces.

                        Having built a trusting relationship with you
                        over a number of sessions, the psychotherapist,
                        who may or may not be medically qualified,
                        focuses on any victim-type negation and helps
                        you to destroy old blockages and to find new
                        openings and faith in yourself.

What doctors think   Doctors usually approve of the use of humanistic psychology therapy.

HYDROTHERAPY

See also Water Therapy

Origins   A truly ancient therapy, the benefits of hydrotherapy were probably first noted when primitive humans appreciated the therapeutic effect of water on their aching body and limbs. Certainly the ancient Romans were fond of their baths; the ancient Greeks, their hot-water springs. The ancient Chinese and Indians were also appreciative of the healing power of water, and spas and vapor baths enjoyed great popularity in Europe. Hydrotherapy is now usually regarded as a part of naturopathy.

What it is   The main forms of hydrotherapy treatment consist of baths (cold, hot, and mineral), compresses (hot and cold), inhalation therapy (steam), physiotherapy in warm water, sitz baths, spray jets and showers, steam baths, and wrapping sheets (hot and cold).

Hydrotherapy is believed to promote self-healing. Its many forms include soaking in a hot bath to sweat out impurities, relax muscles, and ease pain; having a cold bath to treat inflammation and circulation problems; sitting in sitz baths (two side-by-side basins, with a ledge to sit on, filled with hot and cold water to hip level) to treat discomforts such as hemorrhoids and cystitis; wrapping wet clothes around various parts of the body to ease aches, fevers, muscular strains, and pain and to remove toxins; applying hot and cold compresses for stiff muscles and sports injuries, such as sprains; taking alternate hot and cold showers to treat circulation problems, headaches, swelling, and inflammation; having a steam bath, vapor bath, Turkish bath, or sauna to sweat out impurities; sitting in whirlpools to benefit circulation and fluid-retention problems; inhalation to help clear cold symptoms, such as a blocked nose; and receiving physiotherapy in warm water to strengthen weakened muscles.

What it is used for

Hydrotherapy is used for acne; adenoidal infection and inflammation; anemia; anxiety; arthritis; asthma; back pain; bedwetting; blood pressure (high); bronchitis; bruises; bursitis; catarrh; chicken pox; chronic fatigue syndrome; circulation problems; colitis; constipation; cramps; croup; cystitis; depression; fever; fissures; fluid retention; gallstones; gout; headaches; heat rash; hemorrhoids; hyperactivity; incontinence; infertility; inflammation; insomnia; irritable bowel syndrome; joint inflammation; lumbago; measles; menopausal problems; menstrual problems; migraines; muscle weakness; nervous disorders; neuralgia; obesity; panic attacks; psoriasis; rheumatism; sciatica; sleep disorders; sports injuries; stress; tension; throat problems; tiredness; ulcers; vertigo; water retention; wheezing; and whooping cough.

What doctors think

Doctors do recommend hydrotherapy for sports injuries such as sprains, or when suggested by an osteopath, chiropractor, or physiotherapist. These exceptions aside, and although they appreciate the relaxing effect of a warm bath or a foot bath, and the benefits of steam inhalation, doctors remain reserved in their attitude toward hydrotherapy and seem particularly doubtful about the benefits of hot-and-cold treatments.

Warning

If you are allergic to iodine, beware of treatments that include seaweed or seaweed extracts.

Sudden and extreme changes in water temperature can shock the system, resulting in blood pressure problems and fainting. People with heart conditions should consult their family doctor before starting hydrotherapy.

Cold baths and spray treatments for children or people with heart conditions should only be undertaken with full supervision of a specialist.

HYPNOTHERAPY

Origins

Ancient Greek priests and healers used hypnotism for physical and mental ills. In more recent times the Austrian doctor Anton Mesmer—from whose name come our words *mesmerize* and *mesmerism*—was hounded by medical authorities when he achieved fame by putting on public displays of hypnotism. More recently still, Scottish surgeon James Braid used the Greek word *hypnos,* meaning sleep, to describe the trances that he induced in his

patients when they were about to undergo surgery.
As anesthetics and painkilling drugs
improved and became more widely available,
hypnotism lost some of its former glory. It has
recently enjoyed a resurgence of interest.

What it is   Hypnotism induces a trancelike state that hovers
between a day-dream state of mind and sleep.
The conscious mind is thought to be sufficiently
relaxed by hypnotherapy to allow the practitioner
to make contact with the unconscious mind and
bring about positive physical and mental changes
of attitude at a deeper level of consciousness.

Hypnotherapy has achieved significant
recognition for its ability to ameliorate
apprehension, as brought on by a visit to the
dentist, and to act as an effective painkiller. It is
also noted for its success in helping people with
a history of anxiety states, psychosomatic
illnesses, phobias, and stress-related problems.

What it is   Hypnotherapy is used in the treatment of
used for   addiction; alcoholism; allergies; amnesia; anorexia;
anxiety; arthritis; back pain; bedwetting; bulimia;
pain during childbirth; chronic fatigue syndrome;
claustrophobia; colitis; depression; fear;
flatulence; forgetfulness; gout; hay fever;
hyperventilation; hysteria; insomnia; irritable
bowel syndrome; jet lag; menstrual problems;
migraines; mood swings; nervous disorders; pain;
panic attacks; phobias; psychosomatic illnesses;
sciatica; sexual problems; shock; skin disorders;
smoking; snoring; stammering; stress; and warts.

What doctors think

Some dentists and doctors are also qualified hypnotherapists, and many believe that hypnotic trances can be used as a simple pain-relief procedure and for the treatment of some common ailments and disorders.

Others express doubt about what actually happens in hypnotic trances and are concerned that memories and thoughts might be "planted" by the hypnotherapist to produce effects the hypnotherapist or patient wants.

Warning

Hypnotherapy can be dangerous if used inexpertly.

IRIDOLOGY

Origins

The story goes that a Hungarian doctor, Ignatz von Peczeley (1826–1911) stumbled upon iridology in his childhood when caring for a wounded owl. He noticed that a black line in the iris of the owl's eye changed gradually to white marks around a black dot as the owl recovered. Later, as a doctor, he noticed that similar marks appeared at the same position on the iris in patients suffering from the same illness.

After he published his discovery, the news traveled throughout Europe and, by the early 1900s, had reached the United States.

In the 1950s, American physician Bernard Jensen, among others, produced a detailed chart that linked parts of the body to specific areas of the iris.

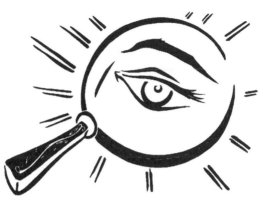

What it is

Iridology is diagnosis through the observation of markings and changes on the iris. The iris is divided into areas that are linked to specific bodily parts and functions, and then into six zones related to the stomach, intestines, blood and lymph systems, glands and organs, muscles and skeleton, and skin and elimination functions.

According to what was "reflected" in a particular area or zone of the iris—for example, a change, such as a new white mark or dark mark—the iridologist can spot early warning signs of trouble or diagnose an existing problem and prescribe appropriate action. Many iridologists do not treat the disorder themselves but suggest a complementary therapy. If serious illness is observed, you will be advised to consult your doctor.

What it is used for

Some people refuse to undergo what they regard as invasive and harmful diagnostic techniques, such as X rays, biopsies, and blood tests, preferring to place their faith in iridology as an alternative for diagnosing possible health problems or checking on the general state of their health.

Complementary practitioners commonly use iridology as an analytical complement to other therapies, such as homeopathy, acupuncture, and herbal medicine.

What doctors think
Although most orthodox doctors make a point of noting when their patients' eyes are dull or overbright, few are prepared to accept iridology as a diagnostic technique, and many worry that treatment for serious illnesses will be unnecessarily delayed.

JIN SHIN DO

See Acupressure

KINESIOLOGY

Origins
George Goodhart discovered kinesiology when he was treating a patient who was suffering from pains in his legs. Puzzled as to why he was achieving such good pain-relieving results when massaging the patient's *fascia lata* (the muscle that runs from hip to knee), but not when massaging other muscles, Goodhart started to match pressure points, pinpointed by osteopath Frank Chapman, to sets of related muscles. He discovered that the pressure point for the *fascia lata* was the only one that lay directly over the muscle.

Continuing the work of a second osteopath, Terence J. Bennet, who had claimed that the circulation of blood to various organs could be dramatically improved by gently touching pressure points on the patient's skull, Goodhart noticed that a few seconds of this fingertip action also strengthened specific muscles. Puzzled by this, he decided to study acupuncture and, having decided that there *are* common energy channels, or meridians, for both organs and muscles, kinesiology was born.

What it is

Kinesiology is a series of major muscle group tests that locate weakness in specific muscles. The findings act as an early alarm to possible health problems or as a way of diagnosing an existing problem. The kinesiologist's painless fingertip pressure tests determine which muscles are working properly and which are weak and working inefficiently. The next step is to establish what is causing the problem and what is needed for correction.

Kinesiologists work on the principle that toxins collect in tissues around pressure points, giving rise to tenderness and discomfort and to ailments that further mar the efficient working of related muscles.

Kinesiologists also claim that their muscle tests are able to spot muscle weakness caused by food allergies, mineral and vitamin deficiencies, and the stagnation of body fluids, which hinders the workings of the lymphatic system and blood flow.

Once the problem is spotted, the kinesiologist uses his or her fingertips to massage the appropriate pressure points on the body or scalp to revitalize the flow of energy, to reestablish a healthy balance, and to disperse toxins.

What it is used for   Kinesiology is used to alleviate allergies; back pain; catarrh; colds; depression; headaches; indigestion; mineral and vitamin deficiencies; muscle weakness; neck pain; sciatica; tension; and tiredness.

What doctors think   The general view is that there has been insufficient scientific research for orthodox doctors to give kinesiology validity as an effective complementary therapy.

MACROBIOTIC DIET THERAPY

See Diet Therapies

MASSAGE

See also Acupressure, Aromatherapy, Kinesiology, Osteopathy, Physiotherapy, Reflexology, Shiatsu

Origins   Massage is known to have been practiced in Middle and Far Eastern countries since about 3,000 B.C., and in ancient Greece where Hippocrates himself recommended a daily massage for the easing of stiffness and pain in joints.

In more recent times, Per Henrik Ling, a Swedish gymnast, popularized a muscle and joint massage system that became known as Swedish massage. An American, George Downing, further popularized massage as a holistic means of helping people to relieve the physical, mental, and emotional tensions of everyday life.

What it is   It is claimed that massage improves physical, mental, and emotional health by dispersing everyday strains and tensions and bringing about a general feeling of relaxation, stability, and well-being. The aims of massage are to relax and relieve the body (physically, mentally, and emotionally); to mobilize stiff joints; to improve blood, muscular, and nervous systems; to help the digestive system to function efficiently; to encourage the disposal of waste from the body; and to aid the prevention and recovery of minor soft-tissue problems.

There are seven main types of massage: effleurage, friction, percussion, pétrissage, connective-tissue techniques, neuromuscular techniques, and stretching techniques. The first four form the basis of Swedish massage.

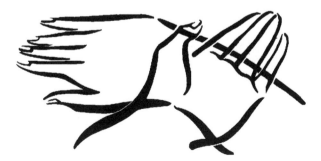

Effleurage

Effleurage offers slow, rhythmic, light- and deep-pressure fingertip, hand, knuckle, and thumbs massage strokes. It is often used in conjunction with aromatherapy oils by aromatherapists.

Friction

Friction massage uses fingertips, thumb pads, and the heels of the hand in small, circular pressure movements to free stiff and locked joints, improve circulation, and treat damaged or strained ligaments and tendons.

Percussion

As its name suggests, percussion is a vigorous but painless drumming massage in which the sides of the hands deliver fast, rhythmic chops to well-padded parts of the body, such as the back, buttocks, and thighs.

Pétrissage

Pétrissage movements are rather like kneading dough. The hands grasp, squeeze, roll, and release whole sections of muscles. The intention of the massage is to improve circulation and to relax contracted muscles.

Connective-tissue techniques

Connective tissue binds muscles and tendons to each other and to bone. Connective-tissue techniques aim to enhance circulation through the connective tissue and thus aid the healing process.

Neuromuscular techniques

Neuromuscular massage works on the interaction between nerves and muscles. Pressure is applied to reflex points in the same way as is used in acupressure.

Stretching techniques

Stretching techniques are techniques used to ease tension in the muscle fibers and, sometimes, to work on muscle adhesions. The practitioner can provide the stretch to the muscle with or without the active assistance of the patient.

What it is used for

It is claimed that, in general, massage improves physical, mental and emotional health by dispersing everyday stresses and bringing about a feeling of relaxation, stability, and well-being.

Success is claimed for treating anxiety; arthritis; asthma; back pain; catarrh; circulation problems; constipation; cramps; depression; digestion problems; exhaustion; fibrositis; fluid retention; foot problems; gout; grief; headaches; hip disorders; hyperactivity; insomnia; jet lag; joint problems; lumbago; menopausal problems; migraines; mood swings; neck pain; nervous disorders; neuralgia; pain; palpitations; panic attacks; postnatal depression; premenstrual tension; rheumatism; schizophrenia; sciatica; shock; sinus problems; sleep disorders; sports injuries; stress; teeth grinding; tennis elbow; and tiredness.

What doctors think

In general, doctors respect and recommend massage for its ability to ease aches and pains, stress, and to bring about relaxation. They are not as approving when it is used for diseases they believe would be better treated by conventional drugs, medicine, or surgery. Some doctors prefer to recommend a physiotherapist for general and sports-injury massage.

Warning

Massage is considered unsuitable for people suffering from phlebitis, thrombosis, varicose veins, or feverish conditions.

MEDITATION

See also Ta'i Chi Ch'uan, Zen Garden Therapy, Zen Therapy

Origins

Meditation has been practiced for thousands of years in India and Asia as a way to reach spiritual enlightenment through personal transformation. There have been many great teachers of meditation. A person who becomes self-realized through meditation and other spiritual practices is considered to be at the zenith of her or his physical, mental, emotional, and spiritual development and is considered to have achieved a spiritual state of union—unity with everything and everyone.

In the 1960s, the Maharishi Mahesh Yogi attracted countless western devotees to

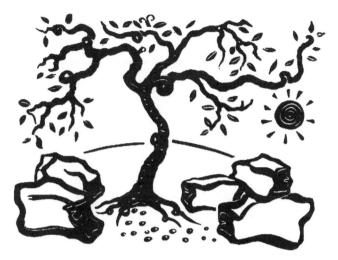

transcendental meditation. Since then there has been great interest in the practice of meditation; even the Christian church has reminded its congregation that various forms of meditation have long been practiced by its religious orders.

What it is   Meditation, usually by focusing the mind on a mantra (spiritual word) or uplifting sentence, is intended to elevate a person above everyday anxieties and distractions and transcend limitations that impede the natural flow of energy and abilities.

Research has shown that meditation slows physiological activity and quiets brain activity.

People usually begin by meditating for ten minutes a day, gradually increasing to twenty or thirty minutes a day, either alone or in a group.

**What it is
used for**   Meditation is used to treat anxiety; asthma;
blood pressure (high); bronchitis; chest
complaints; circulation problems; fears; heart
disease; insomnia; menopausal problems;
muscular tension; panic attacks; phobias; shock;
sleep disorders; stress; tension; and wheezing.

**What doctors
think**   Many doctors are impressed by research showing
that during meditation, breathing, brain activity,
and heart and pulse rate slow and that, as a result
of being in a more relaxed frame of mind, people
are better equipped to cope with everyday stress.

     They are also impressed by patients who
claim that since starting to meditate regularly
they suffer from fewer common ailments and
illnesses.

Warning   Meditation is essentially for people of sound
mind. It is not recommended for people with a
history of mental illness.

MEGAVITAMIN THERAPY

Origins   Linus Pauling, an American biochemist,
popularized his vitamin health therapy in the
book *Vitamin C and the Common Cold*. Before that,
however, two other Americans, Dr. Abraham
Hoffer and Dr. Humphry Osmond, were
successfully treating schizophrenia with high
doses of vitamin B3.

What it is   As the word *mega* implies, the therapy consists of
taking huge doses of vitamins as a self-help

procedure to promote good health, stave off infections, and treat common ailments and illnesses.

Pauling coined the term *orthomolecular medicine* to describe the art of establishing the right level of vitamins and minerals needed to preserve and restore a person's good health at the cellular level; individual needs vary greatly.

What it is used for

Because most illnesses, they emphasize, are linked to metabolic abnormalities caused by a lack of specific vitamins, megavitamin practitioners are convinced that megavitamin therapy can aid most illnesses, including acne; addiction; alcoholism; anemia; chronic fatigue syndrome; depression; nervous disorders; panic attacks; pimples; premenstrual tension; smoking; and viral infections.

Megavitamin therapy is also recommended for counteracting the side effects of orthodox drug treatments, including cancer treatments

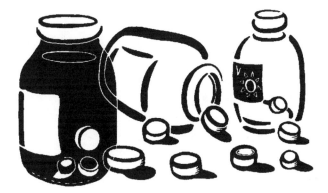

such as chemotherapy. Likewise, it is recommended for people who suffer a vitamin deficiency because of poor appetite during prolonged illness, and for people who seem unable to absorb sufficient vitamins even when their diet is considered well balanced.

Since Linus Pauling first treated schizophrenia with vitamins, the field of orthomolecular psychiatry has expanded to include people with psychiatric problems, such as manic-depressive illness, hyperactivity, and alcohol and drug addiction.

What doctors think

Although there is much research published in mainstream scientific journals, your doctor may have doubts about this particular therapy.

Warning

Although this is regarded as a self-help therapy, it is essential to seek qualified advice before taking large doses of vitamins, which can cause uncomfortable and dangerous side effects if abused. Overdosing on vitamin A, for example, can cause anemia in adults and swellings over bones in children; overdosing on vitamin D can cause hypertension and muscle weakness. For the same reason, ongoing checkups are vital.

MENTAL IMAGING AND RELAXATION

See Visualization Therapy

METAMORPHIC TECHNIQUE

Origins

Robert St. John, a British naturopath, extended his use of reflexology (see page 124 for explanation of this method) to concentrate on the reflex areas relating to the spine. These areas, he became convinced, could tell us much about a person's physical and psychological prebirth development.

St. John believed that both physical and psychological characteristics develop in the womb, and he was convinced that health problems would continue to recur—even after treatment—unless people could be helped to "appreciate" the presence of problems that stemmed from his or her prenatal stage of development and to receive treatment to help correct them.

What it is

Practitioners of the metamorphic technique use circular, sometimes called "vibrating," finger movements to manipulate the bony ridge running along the inner side of the foot, the big toe, and the ankle. The outside edge down the thumb to the wrist, and a central line from the top of the head to the base of the skull and then along the bony ridge on each side toward the ears are also massaged. Practitioners regard themselves as catalysts who, through "acceptance" of whatever is found during a session, allow the person being treated to connect with his or her self-healing powers.

What it is used for
The metamorphic technique will aid anyone who wants help for a long-term or recurring health problem. Practitioners claim it is particularly useful for people born with physical or mental disabilities, such as Down's syndrome, and success has been claimed for children with autism.

What doctors think
Many doctors dismiss the metamorphic technique; others say they are reserving judgment until claims are either substantiated or invalidated by research.

MUSIC THERAPY

Origins
Music, both making it and listening to it, has been recognized as having healing qualities since ancient times. Recent studies confirm its usefulness as a therapy.

What it is
Music practitioners—who need to be trained musicians with a university-level qualification and postgraduate training from a recognized therapy

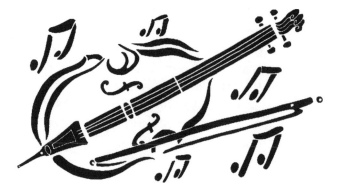

center—primarily use the therapy of making music to unlock or reveal what are often deeply based emotional blocks. It is thought that if these are left unexpressed, they may give rise to physical ailments, mental problems, and stress.

The idea is to help people make sounds and music, through a range of instruments or through singing, until they reach a phase in which they are able to express long-repressed negative feelings, such as resentment, anger, jealousy, hatred, and fury, or repressed positive sensations, such as pleasure and joy.

The role of the practitioner is to encourage, to observe, to ask appropriate questions to draw out need-revealing responses and, on the basis of this information, to assess the psychotherapeutic process and ongoing therapy program.

People are encouraged to choose their own methods of making music. They do not need to be musical, in the sense of having experience or knowledge of music. The therapy is said to work however crude the music.

What it is used for

Children and adults with physical or learning disabilities, or who are mentally or emotionally disturbed or ill, can benefit from music therapy, as can the elderly—especially those in care centers—for whom this therapy can provide a valuable means of communication.

Success also has been claimed for those with autism, breathing problems, communication problems, nervous disorders, schizophrenia, speech problems, and stress.

Autism

Autistic children are withdrawn, living in a world of their own. They rarely respond to expressions of affection, including those given by their families, and although given to explosive behavior they do not communicate with others through speech, facial expressions, or other means.

Parents have been amazed by how music therapy has helped to arouse responses in their autistic children, to soothe them, and to reduce violent outbursts.

Nervous Disorders

Music therapy can markedly reduce anxiety and panic attacks in people suffering from nervous disorders, increasing their sense of self-worth and enabling them to express deeply repressed anguish and fears.

Schizophrenia

Music, both making and listening to it, is claimed to have helped some schizophrenics to be much less at the mercy of delusions and to gain some control over their lives.

Stress

Making and listening to music can be a great mood changer and quite therapeutic for easing the stresses of everyday life and their associated health problems.

What doctors think   Noting how music can produce a change of mood and soothe or raise the spirits, most doctors readily acknowledge it as a healing force. They increasingly recommend music therapy as a health-promoting treatment, especially for people coping with physical difficulties and for people dealing with emotional and mental issues.

NATURAL CHILDBIRTH

See Special Needs section, page 215

NATURAL FAMILY PLANNING

See Special Needs section, page 211

NATUROPATHY

Origins   In the early days, naturopathy was known as "nature cure." Its origins are usually attributed to Hippocrates who, two thousand years ago, stressed that the key to good health is to live as naturally and moderately as possible. Certainly, he approached healing with admirable "first do no harm," let-the-body-heal-itself principles.

Others believe that its origins are as old as the human race; that it came into being with the first human to pick up a leaf to cover an injured leg, to find a root to chew, to use a pool of water to ease an aching foot or, through watching an injured animal, to observe the innate healing wisdom that animals display.

What it is

The main approach of naturopathy is, as its name suggests, natural, using anything and everything that will help the body to heal itself by reestablishing balance where there is imbalance. Its essential work is to establish the cause of a breakdown in health and then to alleviate, rather than suppress, symptoms.

Practitioners believe in retaining positive attitudes and as natural a lifestyle as possible amid the unnaturalness of the modern world. Their holistic approach concentrates on each person as an individual with individual needs.

What it is used for

Naturopathy is regarded as a complement to orthodox medicine and is used to help treat acid stomach; acne; addiction; adenoids; alcoholism; anemia; angina; anorexia; anxiety; arteries (hardening of); arthritis; asthma; bee stings; bites; blood pressure (high and low); blisters; boils; bronchitis; bruising; bunions; bursitis; cataracts; catarrh; chicken pox; chilblains; chronic fatigue syndrome; cold sores; colds; colitis; conjunctivitis; constipation; corns; coughs; cramps; croup; cystitis; dandruff; diarrhea; dizziness; dysentery; eczema; emphysema; epilepsy; eyestrain; fever; flatulence; fluid retention; fungal infections; gallstones; genital herpes; glandular fever; gout; hangover; hay fever; headaches; hemorrhoids; hives; hyperactivity; hypoglycemia; hypothermia; impetigo; incontinence; indigestion; infertility; influenza; irritable bowel syndrome; itching; laryngitis; measles; menopausal problems; morning sickness; mumps; nausea and vomiting; neuralgia; nose bleeds; obesity; osteoporosis; panic attacks; pimples; premenstrual tension; shingles; sneezing; stings; stress; sty; sunburn; sweating; tension; thrush; tonsillitis; ulcers (leg, mouth, and peptic); varicose veins; viral infections; wheezing; whooping cough; and worms.

What doctors think   The response of doctors to naturopathy, as a whole, is positive. Some doubts are expressed when less-accepted complementary therapies are recommended by naturopaths, and some doctors question the wisdom of delaying orthodox treatment for certain conditions.

NUTRITIONAL THERAPIES

See Diet Therapies

OILS THERAPY

See Aromatherapy

OSTEOPATHY

See also Chiropractic

Origins

Andrew Taylor Still (1828–1917) founded osteopathy after becoming disillusioned with orthodox drug treatments. With his knowledge of human anatomy, he was convinced that manipulation could correct physical misalignment and complement the body's powers of self-healing.

What it is

Osteopaths believe that the true alignment of the human skeleton—the body's main framework—allows us to move and function easily and efficiently and that misalignment is responsible for discomfort, pain, common ailments, and serious health problems.

Osteopaths use their hands for massage and gentle repetitive manipulation of joints, giving particular attention to the vertebrae and the discs between them. In addition to treating mechanical problems and helping the body to work more efficiently, the release of physical stress through osteopathy is said to help people suffering from tension headaches and breathing problems such as asthma.

What it is used for

Osteopathy is used in the treatment of arthritis; asthma; back pain; cramps; fibrositis; foot problems; gout; headaches; joint problems; lumbago; neck pain; neuralgia; osteoarthritis; postural problems; pregnancy (lower-back problems); sciatica; slipped disc; snoring; sports injuries (to ligaments, muscles, and joints); teeth grinding; tennis elbow; and varicose veins.

What doctors think   A very slow acceptance has given way to approval of osteopathy as an effective way to treat skeletal problems, and doctors now often refer patients to osteopaths. There is less acceptance for its use in treating nonskeletal problems, such as headaches. Many orthodox doctors are now registered osteopaths.

PHOBIA THERAPIES

See Art Therapy, Behavioral Therapy, Counseling, Homeopathy, Hypnotherapy, Psychotherapy

PHYSIOTHERAPY

Origins   Physiotherapy was established by four nurses and midwives who wanted to regularize the practice of massage, or "medical rubbing," in the late nineteenth century.

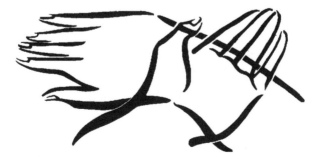

What it is Perhaps the best known of all the complementary
therapies, physiotherapy is treatment by physical
means including massage, manipulation, exercise
and movement, heat and cold, and light and
other electrophysical agencies. Essentially a
hands-on profession, it uses touch as a diagnostic
and treatment tool as well as a psychological
support. It is an independent profession working
closely with other professions in health,
education, and social care.

What it is Physiotherapy is used to treat a host of common
used for ailments and illnesses, including injuries of all
kinds (for example, those caused by car
accidents, accidents at home, and in sports); joint
disorders (such as arthritis); neck, back, and joint
pain (such as lumbago, sciatica, and repetitive
strain injuries); mobility problems of all kinds;
muscle weakness and wastage; and respiratory
problems (such as asthma, bronchitis, and
emphysema).

Physiotherapy is in common use in day-care
centers, hospitals, special schools, and for
treating long-term patients and age-related
problems. It is regularly used for children and
adults with physical, emotional, and mental
disabilities and for people confined to care
centers, hospitals, or wheelchairs.

What doctors Doctors give physiotherapy unreserved approval
think as an essential adjunct to orthodox procedures.

PHYTOTHERAPY

A recently introduced word, phytotherapy describes the work of medical herbalists who harness the healing power of plants and herbs.

POLARITY THERAPY

Origins

Randolph Stone, an Austrian-born American, trained in chiropractic, naturopathy, and osteopathy, then went on to study eastern healing systems, including acupuncture, ayurvedic medicine, and yoga. Seeking to understand why certain illnesses recurred after initially responding to massage-type treatment, Stone devised a system based on "life energy" principles, and polarity therapy came into being.

What it is

The life energy that Stone came to believe governed a person's physical, mental, emotional, and spiritual well-being, could, he reasoned, become blocked by bad habits, such as poor diet, and by harmful behavior, resulting in stresses that take their toll on all the body's functions.

Believing that good health depends on a polarity, or a balancing, of the life force, Stone used his knowledge of eastern and western healing systems to devise a method of polarity healing that would rebalance and unblock the body's vital energy, promoting the body's natural self-healing powers. Once the balance was reestablished, good health would be restored.

Stone's polarity therapy involves five energy centers, based on the five basic elements, which are said to govern main areas of the body:

ether—throat and ears

air—heart, chest, shoulders, skin, kidneys, lungs, and colon

fire—digestive organs, eyes, gall bladder, liver, pancreas, spleen, and sympathetic nervous system

water—bladder, pelvis, endocrine system, generative system, heart, and lymphatic system

earth—neck, colon, knees, elimination, intestines, and skeletal system

Polarity, Stone said, could be reestablished through four health-promoting techniques: bodywork or therapeutic touch; awareness skills; diet and nutrition; and stretching exercises.

Manipulation and Bodywork

The polarity practitioner uses three types of touch: positive (energizing, stimulating); neutral (light, balancing); and negative (deep, dissipating) to release and polarize blocked energy.

Awareness Skills

The practitioner is trained in skills that allow the interaction of the body and mind to become fuller and deeper.

Diet and Nutrition

Health-building or cleansing diet procedures can help detoxify the system, freeing the life-giving energy. The practitioner carefully assesses each person individually, as no one procedure is correct for everyone.

Polarity Stretching Exercises

Stretching exercises release stagnation and help people to continue and maintain the healing process.

On your first visit you will be asked for details of your medical history, and the practitioner will assess your physical structure and energy patterns.

What it is used for

Practitioners are convinced that polarity can help anybody, but stress that its success depends on an individual's full cooperation and commitment to change. They emphasize that the therapy concentrates on restoring the balance of the body's vital energies rather than focusing on the symptoms of illness and disease.

What doctors think

When doctors break down the various components of polarity therapy into orthodox terms of a system based on bodywork, counseling, diet, and exercise, they are usually receptive.

POSTURAL THERAPY

See Alexander Technique

PRESSURE POINT THERAPIES

See Acupressure, Acupuncture, Aromatherapy, Chiropractic, Massage, Osteopathy, Physiotherapy, Shiatsu, Zone Therapy

PRIMAL SCREAM THERAPY

See also Rebirthing Therapy

Origins

Primal scream therapy had its beginnings in the ideas of Arthur Janov, an American psychiatrist who was influenced by Sigmund Freud and Wilhelm Reich. Alice Miller, a Swiss analyst, was in turn influenced by Janov and has written widely about child-rearing practices. Both doctors were influential in the recent work of J. Konrad Stettbacher, a Swiss primal practitioner.

What it is

Primal scream therapy is intended to help people face up to the unfinished business and unfulfilled needs of their babyhood and childhood.

Children tend to feel responsible when bad things happen to them. Rather than see the parent as "bad," they see themselves as wrong or unworthy. This can result in strong feelings of shame and guilt, and a sense of being unlovable.

Janov believed that giving vent to a "primal scream," expressing emotional and mental pain, could heal and, perhaps, free a person from the anguish of his or her babyhood and childhood.

What it is used for

The therapy is aimed at the cause of emotional disorders by releasing the anguish of adults still living in the shadow of babyhood or childhood unfulfillment. This is achieved by resolving conflicts that originated from lack of parental love and affection; from being undermined when seemingly failing to live up to parents' impossibly high standards and expectations; and from being physically or sexually abused by a parent and feeling somehow responsible, and terrified of losing him or her by revealing the secret.

Primal scream therapy can be carried out in several ways. Some practitioners favor an intensive phase of therapy, perhaps with weekend follow-ups; others believe that if childhood experiences are to be uncovered in a meaningful way and worked through safely, patients need the support of or regular ongoing contact with the therapist.

What doctors think

Doctors have mixed reactions to primal scream therapy, but do admit that people can continue to suffer from babyhood and childhood experiences. They usually stop short of including birth experiences, however.

Warning

The therapy can be traumatic if not enough ongoing support is offered.

PSYCHOTHERAPY

See also Counseling

Origins   Using what came to be known as psychoanalysis,
Sigmund Freud, the Austrian psychiatrist,
encouraged his patients to relive trauma in order
to free themselves from blocks or repressions
that had created neurotic behavior and nervous
disorders.

Psychotherapy is based on Freud's methods,
but is usually less long term and less time
consuming than psychoanalysis.

What it is   Anybody who has had a session getting things off
their chest to somebody who is a good listener
knows what psychotherapy is. The difference
between a psychotherapist and a friend who is a
good listener is, of course, that the first has
received professional training in how to help
others reveal underlying anxiety, anguish,
communication problems, marital problems, or
neurosis. A psychotherapist draws on his or her
training to offer advice, counseling, or
encouragement.

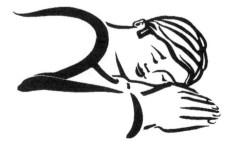

The main difference between counseling and psychotherapy is that counseling is used to assist people to "adjust": to come to terms, for example, with bereavement, divorce, accident shock, and trauma. Psychotherapy, presupposing that something is wrong with the patient, provides more deep-seated, long-term work on the patient's emotional and personality disorders and the need for change or developing new coping strategies.

Psychotherapy can take place on a one-to-one basis or in a group.

The relationship between the psychotherapist and patient needs to be close and trusting. Some people believe that the psychotherapist should be a unisex mother-father substitute, so that the patient can resolve through the relationship problems that stem from his or her relationship with parents or from experiences between babyhood and adolescence.

Psychotherapists, unlike psychiatrists, are not usually medically trained and cannot prescribe orthodox drug or shock treatments. Many people interested in complementary therapies would regard that as an advantage.

What it is used for

Success is claimed for a wide range of symptoms, including depression, anxiety, eating disorders, and physical symptoms. Psychotherapy can help people to come to terms with serious illness and disability. Research has shown that life expectancy for women with breast cancer is longer for those who participate in group psychotherapy.

People expressing themselves through antisocial behavior; experiencing communication and other problems with relationships; struggling with a personality problem; or having problems concerned with emotional, mental, or spiritual disturbance could benefit from psychotherapy.

What doctors think

Doctors today accept that emotional and psychological problems play an important part in physical ailments and serious illness, as well as emotional, mental, and spiritual disorders. They accept that pressure on their own patient-care time leaves insufficient time to concentrate on psychosomatic factors, so they often recommend psychotherapy or counseling for specific disorders.

RADIONICS THERAPY

Origins

The principles of radionics therapy were discovered by an American doctor. As the therapy falls outside the scope of accepted orthodox medicine, it has been carried on and developed by nonmedical practitioners.

What it is

Practitioners of radionics believe that everything and everyone emits energy patterns and that any disharmonies or distortions in the patterns can be identified and measured with the aid of special instruments.

One of the advantages of radionics therapy is that the practitioner does not require the presence of the patient—either for analysis or treatment—and only needs a witness, such as a lock of hair, to act as a link between patient and instrument. The patient fills in a case-history form, which is returned to the practitioner with a lock of hair. The practitioner's analysis will record any malfunctions, infections, injuries, or blockages. The practitioner then seeks the prime or deep cause, and may then advise the patient as to which therapy to use.

What it is used for

Radionics therapy is used to treat allergic conditions; arthritis; asthma; dyslexia; hay fever; hypersensitivity; mental illness; and psychological states. Animals also respond well to this treatment.

What doctors think

Most doctors are seriously skeptical of any healing that works at a distance.

RAW FOOD DIET THERAPY

See Diet Therapies

REBIRTHING THERAPY

See also Primal Scream Therapy

Origins

Some psychologists believe the process of birth can have life-long effects. They assert that the birthing process is traumatic, due in part to the terror of emerging from a warm womb where every need has been met into a cold, vast world filled with stimuli the infant does not understand.

What it is   In rebirthing therapy, also called *conscious-connected breathing* or *vivation,* a therapist guides a person through breathing exercises that allow the person to relive his or her birth in order to release some of the anxiety and fears that originated there.

What it is used for   By encouraging people to express repressed trauma—which, with nowhere to go, results in emotional blocks and more serious emotional problems and mental disorders—rebirthing is believed to bring healing to physical, mental, and emotional disorders.

What doctors think   While accepting that many of our emotional, mental, and spiritual attitudes derive from babyhood and childhood experiences, and that unresolved trauma takes its toll on adult life, doctors are, as a whole, less accepting of rebirthing therapy than primal scream therapy (see page 118).

REFLEXOLOGY

Origins   This ancient pressure-point therapy is thought to have been brought to the west in the early 1900s by William Fitzgerald, an American ear, nose, and throat specialist. He called his system *zone therapy* (see page 147). His ideas were taken up by the American therapist Eunice Ingham, who concentrated her efforts on one zone, the feet.

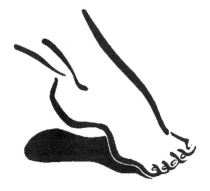

What it is   Reflexology is a system of applying massage to
major reflex areas on the soles of the feet, which
are said to mirror, or reflect, the condition of
other parts of the body, such as the neck, kidney,
and gall bladder. The reflexologist locates tender
spots—the tenderness being an indication of
illness in the associated part of the body—and
treats the problem by applying special massage
techniques to the appropriate area of the foot.
Some practitioners, using the Morrell method
(see below), visually inspect the feet to obtain
information and may use only the lightest
exploratory touch.

    The right foot is said to reflect the right side
of the body; the left, the left side of the body. As
in many therapies, it is believed that health
problems result from blockages in natural energy
channels. Massage heals the body by reopening
the channels, allowing the natural flow.

    It is important to seek out a fully qualified
reflexologist. At your first visit, the practitioner
will review your medical history and make an
initial examination of your feet, noting any

existing conditions, such as bunions, which are thought to interfere with the blood supply. Then, using the side and end of the right or left thumb (for the Morrell method, the pads of the thumb and fingers are used), the reflexologist will feel for any tenderness on either foot. In addition to paying specific attention to this area or areas, the practitioner will massage all the reflex areas on both feet.

What it is used for

Reflexology is used for a wide range of common ailments and serious illnesses, including agoraphobia; arthritis; asthma; athlete's foot; back pain; blood pressure (high); breast problems; bronchitis; catarrh; claustrophobia; constipation; cystitis; eczema; hypoglycemia; indigestion; jaundice; joint problems; kidney complaints; lumbago; menstrual problems; migraines; neck pain; rheumatism; sinus problems; stress; and strokes.

What doctors think

While many doctors think that nothing but good can come from a comforting foot massage, others feel that there has been insufficient research and clinical trials to back up practitioners' claims.

Warning

Reflexology is not recommended for people suffering from psychotic conditions or thrombosis, notifiable diseases, or for pregnant women.

REICHIAN THERAPY

Origins
Wilhelm Reich, an Austrian psychiatrist, started off a devotee of Freud. Later he had a change of mind and heart about Freudianism and developed his own methods, now known as Reichian therapy.

Reich also proposed controversial theories concerning the repression of "orgone energy," energy associated with sexual orgasm. He believed that repression of orgone energy results in emotional disturbance and psychological problems. He invented an orgone accumulator box, in which his patients were asked to sit to recharge their orgone energy. Orgone therapy was vigorously attacked by both psychologists and scientists.

Reich's career ended when he was jailed for selling equipment and continuing to publish theories that had been prohibited by U.S. medical authorities. Since his death in prison in 1957, his methods have regained some devotees, and developed into the field of bioenergetics (see page 42).

What it is
The Reichian therapist encourages the person to become aware of how his or her "body armoring"—the posture and muscular tensions—is reflected in the way he or she breathes and how it reflects his or her feelings and frame of mind. The practitioner then uses physical movements and postural adjustments, including manipulation, to help free repressions and release tension.

What doctors think　Both doctors and scientists remain skeptical of Reichian therapy, and await scientific substantiation of claims by people who say they have been helped and by practitioners.

Rogerian Therapy

Origins　Carl Rogers, one of the chief pioneers of humanistic psychology therapy (see page 86), believed that physical, mental, and emotional problems arise when people lose touch with themselves and become overdependent on the approval of others and overinfluenced by what others decide is acceptable behavior.

What it is　Rogers' therapy, which became known as Rogerian therapy or client-centered therapy, aims to decrease the negative aspects of overdependence on others and to increase the positive aspects of self-dependence. Self-reliance is nurtured through the belief that, whatever the genetic, family, environmental, and social influences around you, you are in charge of your own life. Rogerian therapy is not about increasing selfishness at the expense of others; the aim is to use the ensuing greater sense of self-fulfillment for the collective benefit of yourself and others.

The practitioner usually begins by establishing the main problem area, then, by listening and gently guiding, encourages you to understand that ultimately only *you* can free and fulfill yourself.

What it is
used for   Rogerian therapy is used to counteract a "victim" mentality, the belief that one is solely the helpless product of conditioning. Success is claimed for anxiety, stress-related and emotional problems, and for people who are conscious that negative attitudes and a sense of helplessness are marring their relationships and their life.

What doctors
think   Rogerian therapy is regarded as a successful therapy with healthful, positive consequences.

ROLFING

Origins   Ida Rolf, an American biochemist, theorized that the body's posture and muscular tensions were held in place by connective tissue. Connective tissues assume their shape, she reasoned, in response to injuries we have suffered, habits we have adopted, and the force of gravity. Rolf conceived a system of manipulation and education designed to restore the body's physical balance.

What it is   Rolf's system has evolved into a series of ten sessions during which the practitioner works gently but deeply, with the hands, to untangle the web of connective tissues. During the sessions, the client learns to relax and is also helped by making slow, precise movements. Posture begins to improve, and the body's carriage and movement becomes lighter and more responsive. A trusting relationship between practitioner and client is critical, as the bodily

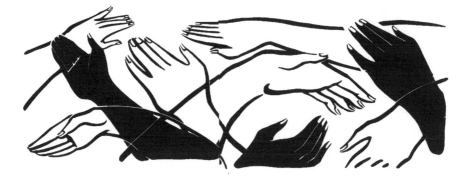

changes take place at a physical and emotional level.

What it is used for
Rolfing is commonly used to combat pain brought about by poor posture or chronic structural imbalance. It is used by dancers and athletes and is compatible with most exercise disciplines; it is also used to correct postural attitudes of the body brought about by emotional tension.

What doctors think
Doctors consider Rolfing a useful tool for learning about the body, but do not believe it should be used instead of standard medical treatment.

SHIATSU

Origins
Shiatsu is a pressure-point massage therapy that has been practiced for centuries. It was developed in Japan to benefit body, mind, and spirit.

What it is   Like acupressure, Shiatsu, which means "finger pressure," employs the fingers, hands, elbows, forearms, and even knees and feet to apply pressure to hundreds of surface points along the body's energy paths, or meridians.

By calming or stimulating hundreds of pressure points, Shiatsu rebalances the electromagnetic forces of the body and releases a flow of energy, life force, which enhances a person's vitality and natural healing powers.

What it is used for   Shiatsu is used to relieve back pain; constipation; diarrhea; headaches; indigestion; insomnia; joint problems; migraines; sports injuries; stress; tension; throat problems; and toothache. It is particularly useful for anything stress related.

Shiatsu is also recommended for convalescence periods and for generally improving circulation and the nervous and immune systems.

What doctors think   Doctors accept Shiatsu as a pain-relieving and relaxing technique, provided the warning below is heeded. Some doctors have Shiatsu practitioners within their practice.

Warning   This therapy should not be used to treat bone fractures, inflamed or injured areas, or slipped discs, or by people taking steroids.

SHIN TAO

See Acupressure

SOUND THERAPY

See also Cymatic Therapy

Origins

The therapeutic qualities of sound have been known since ancient times and have long been used in eastern and western religions and spiritual practices, such as meditation and chanting of prayers (for example, Gregorian chants).

Today's sound therapists believe that sound waves can be directed to specific parts of the body for healing effects.

What it is

Scientific evaluation has established that sound waves can bring relief and healing. Sound waves can work in cooperation with the basic harmonic sound produced by the body's cells and organs. All cells hold a particular note and when these are accumulated together they produce the harmonic sound known as the "H" factor.

The practitioner uses a handheld applicator, and sometimes pads or plates, to transmit sound waves. The sound waves can be generated at many frequencies; the practitioner establishes the condition to be treated and selects the appropriate frequencies.

What it is used for

Sound waves are used for treating, among other conditions, arthritis and allied complaints; bone fractures; migraines; neuralgia; rheumatism; and sports injuries.

What doctors think   There is general agreement by doctors that sound has definite therapeutic qualities and can be emotionally uplifting, but there is a general reluctance to accept the healing claims made for sound therapy.

SOUND WAVE THERAPY

See Cymatic Therapy, Sound Therapy

STRESS THERAPIES

Excessive stress leads to a variety of problems. The main goal of stress management is for sufferers to understand more about the causes, consequences, and effects of stress, and to learn skills to enable them to cope better with problems that arise. The following therapies may help with relaxation or stress management: Aromatherapy, Art Therapy, Autogenic Training Therapy, Behavioral Therapy, Bioenergetics, Counseling, Dance Movement Therapy, Herbal Medicine, Homeopathy, Hypnotherapy, Kinesiology, Massage, Meditation, Naturopathy, Psychotherapy, Reflexology, Sound Therapy, Ta'i Chi Ch'uan Therapy, and Yoga.

TA'I CHI CH'UAN THERAPY

Origins   Ta'i Chi Ch'uan is about four hundred and fifty years old. Its origins lie in Taoist principles

concerned with the need to harmonize with
natural events.

What it is   Ta'i Chi Ch'uan is a Chinese health-enhancement
system for the prevention and treatment of
disease. The literal translation is "supreme
ultimate fist," a reference to its martial arts
applications. It consists of movements linked
together in a continuous stream, which gave rise
to the name "long river boxing."

Ta'i Chi Ch'uan is practiced slowly and
smoothly in a defined pattern and with precise
postural alignment. The mind is focused, with a
strong sense of purpose; this is coupled with a
deep, calm, breathing pattern that is coordinated
with the movements.

Ta'i Chi Ch'uan should be practiced on a
regular basis, preferably in a class, for at least
ninety minutes a week. A skillful, knowledgeable
teacher is essential.

**What it is
used for**   Ta'i Chi Ch'uan accords with the principles of
traditional Chinese medicine; in China it is used
in hospitals for treating chronic disease and
other conditions and has a well-documented
success rate. It is used in the west mainly for
combating stress and stress-related problems. It is
useful for the treatment of arthritis and to aid
recuperation in injury.

**What doctors
think**   Doctors who have some knowledge of Ta'i Chi
Ch'uan are positive about its benefits.

TRAGERWORK

Origins

Milton Trager began developing a technique in 1927 that would help reeducate people to move in ways that effect a more efficient use of body and mind. After becoming a medical doctor in 1955 and working in general medicine and physical rehabilitation for eighteen years, he opened the Trager Institute in 1975.

What it is

Tragerwork is perhaps less a physical therapy than a mental attitude. Tragerwork sessions involve the movement of muscles, limbs, and joints to produce feelings of lightness and freedom. The practitioner uses the hands and mind to communicate these feelings through the patient's tissue to the central nervous system, reawakening a sense of playfulness within the patient.

Following this aided movement, a patient begins lessons in *Mentastics,* or mental gymnastics, exercises intended to integrate mind and body. Mentastics involve simple, dancelike movements intended to bring about feelings of lightness.

TRANSACTIONAL ANALYSIS THERAPY

Origins

Transactional analysis (TA) was developed in the late 1950s by Eric Berne, an American psychiatrist. He had been trained as a Freudian psychoanalyst, and his system retains many of Freud's original ideas. However, in place of the abstract theoretical framework of traditional psychoanalysis, Berne focused on people's observable behavior; in particular he analyzed people's ways of communicating with each other—their everyday *transactions.*

What it is   TA therapy is action oriented; the emphasis is on achieving practical change, not simply on gaining insight.

TA theory suggests that each of us shows three different types of ego state: parent, adult, and child. In the adult ego state, we deal with situations using mature abilities of understanding and problem solving. Sometimes, however—particularly under stress—we may move into a child ego state in which we think, feel, and behave as we did in childhood. Or we may shift to a parent ego state, in which we deal with the world in ways that we learned from our parents or parental figures.

TA practitioners help their clients to become aware of shifts in ego state. The objective of therapy is to gain autonomy, to be able to choose ego states and communication styles flexibly to enhance life and relationships.

What it is used for   TA is notable for its wide range of application; it has been used successfully with many types of personal problems.

What doctors think   The general feeling is that TA therapy can reach a wide cross-section of people and can often bring measurable results in a short time through its emphasis on active change.

VEGANISM

See Diet Therapies

VEGETARIANISM

See Diet Therapies

VISUALIZATION THERAPY

Origins

The conjuring up of healing images is an ancient art, probably as old as the human race, and it was certainly used by witch doctors and by priests in ancient Greece.

Much later, Americans Edmund Jacobson, then Carl Simonton and Stephanie Simonton, then surgeon Bernard Siegel explored and researched visualization therapy. Their findings popularized it as a healing therapy.

What it is

We all know that the images we hold of ourselves can raise and lower self-esteem and affect how we act physically, how we feel emotionally, and how we respond to people and events.

Visualization therapy takes this process a step further. People learn to "see the way to health": how to use positive images to help us feel better about ourselves, other people, and life itself.

Having established the problem, the practitioner usually begins by asking the person to imagine a scene that is related to the problem—any images can be drawn on for this—and to describe what she or he sees. After considering the image together, the practitioner encourages the person to become aware of physical and emotional sensations. Gradually, through the introduction of subtle adjustments to the inner picture, negative aspects give way to positive ones, and healing takes place.

What it is used for

Visualization is used for most physical and emotional problems. Success is claimed for asthma, heart disorders, pain relief, and phobias; as an aid to breathing and relaxation exercises; and as a reliever of stress and tension.

Elderly people have claimed that, with ten minutes a day of visualization therapy, they have achieved greater resistance to illness and that, in general, they lead a more active, happier, and creative life.

What doctors think

Doctors' opinion of visualization therapy depends on what it is being used for. It is regarded as a controversial therapy when used for "treating" serious illnesses, especially those likely to be terminal. It is, however, generally approved of as an aid to relaxation, a better self-image, and stress-related problems.

VITAMIN THERAPY

See Megavitamin Therapy

WATER THERAPY

See also Hydrotherapy

Origins

This is an ancient therapy. The ancient Chinese, Greeks, and Romans often built their temples by hot springs. Hydros, or spas, as they subsequently became known, became very popular in Europe, and their presence was responsible for many resorts becoming fashionable. Natural hot-spring water baths are enjoying a revival at present.

What it is

Water therapy is summed up in the expressions "visiting the spas" or "taking the waters." It is best described as aquatic physiotherapy, a relaxing floating, in soothing, warm mineral water. Soaking is sometimes accompanied by stretches and exercise, and wet-and-hot treatments in beauty therapy rooms.

The expression "taking the waters" came from drinking the water, in addition to getting

into it. Today, the sale of bottled natural-spring mineral waters means that millions of people "take the waters" every day.

What it is used for   Water therapy can help relieve muscle and joint problems, such as arthritis and rheumatism; tension; and stress-related disorders.

What doctors think   Doctors give the curative effects of water therapy their seal of approval.

YIN AND YANG THERAPY

Origins   This Chinese philosophy is so ancient that its origins have been lost. The first known reference, dated about A.D. 200, stems from Chang Chung's work on a yin-yang treatment system for a multitude of symptoms and ills.

What it is   A philosophical concept—common to all aspects of Chinese medicine—is that the perfect balance of the two complementary life forces, yin and

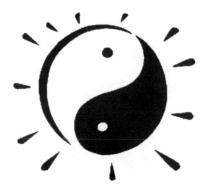

yang, results in good health, and an imbalance results in problems. Yin is a passive, energy-conserving force; yang is a positive, active force.

What it is used for

See the various alternative therapies based on yin and yang principles, including Acupressure, Acupuncture, Macrobiotic Diet Therapy, Shiatsu, Reflexology, and Ta'i Chi Ch'uan Therapy.

YOGA

Origins

Nobody knows how ancient this Indian system is, only that it has been found illustrated on seals dating back over four thousand years.

Yoga was once practiced only by Indian philosophers and yogis, who withdrew from ordinary life to live the life of ascetics. Yoga classes are now available for schoolchildren in India and for millions of people worldwide.

What it is

The word yoga means "union," and in the largest sense of the word means being at one, at complete harmony, with one's self and everything and everybody in creation.

A holistic training system for the benefit of the body, mind, emotions, and spirit, yoga teaches self-control through a series of exercises, levels of breathing, postures, relaxation, and meditation.

Its spiritual aim is to free people from being at the mercy of every passing fancy, distraction, thought or feeling and to enable them to cope with life's everyday problems. The ultimate goal is for each individual to reach his or her full physical, mental, emotional, and spiritual potential for the benefit of humankind.

Patanjali, a great yoga scholar, taught that yoga has eight essential aspects: The first two concern living a moderate, peaceful, harmonious life, shunning excess and avoiding anything that harms others. The second two aspects concern exercises and breathing practices for mental well-being. The remaining four aspects are concerned with learning to detach oneself at will from everyday activities and to achieve a liberated, expansive state in which spiritual transformation allows one to experience the true nature of reality.

Beginning and advanced yoga classes are widely available; sessions usually last between sixty and ninety minutes. Progress depends on regular attendance and a willingness to practice at home. Light, loose clothing is recommended, and one should refrain from eating for at least two hours before practicing.

The many schools of yoga are differentiated by their approach—whether, for example, they place the emphasis on breathing, meditation, posture, relaxation, or spiritual aspects. Individuals need to locate the approach that best suits them.

There are medically trained yoga practitioners who give one-to-one or small-group sessions in which they concentrate on a particular need or problem and develop yoga routines for specific individuals.

What it is
used for

Like other forms of movement, meditation, and relaxation, yoga claims to bring relief from many ailments and diseases, including alcoholism; anxiety; arthritis; asthma; back pain; blood pressure (high) bronchitis; diabetes; heart disease; hemorrhoids; hyperventilation; insomnia; irritable bowel syndrome; menopausal problems; migraines; nerve or muscle disease; obesity; osteoporosis; panic attacks; postnatal depression; premenstrual tension; preparing mothers-to-be for natural childbirth; rheumatism; smoking; stress; and varicose veins.

What doctors
think

Doctors have a mixed reaction toward yoga, ranging from approval for it as a form of exercise beneficial for relaxation, to doubts about it being used for serious conditions. Some doctors have taken part in trials to measure its effects scientifically.

ZEN GARDEN THERAPY

Origins

As old as Zen Buddhism itself, which began in India in the sixth century B.C., Zen gardens are still found in the grounds of Zen Buddhist temples. Among the most famous is Japan's fifteenth-century Ryoan-ji Zen Garden at Kyoto.

What it is

Zen garden therapy is a do-it-yourself aid in the sense that you can create your own garden, harmonious surroundings in which to practice meditation or simply sit and contemplate your inner state of mind and body.

The most important consideration when planning a Zen garden is that it should be essentially harmonious, free of colors, shapes, and textures that clash with each other or distract the attention from meditation or contemplation. A sense of balance, space, and privacy are essential ingredients. Zen gardens usually contain a few large rocks, set off-center; a bonsai-type tree, centered; shrubs as a background; and neatly raked, perfectly level gravel, pea shingle, or very short grass in the foreground. The back of the garden is usually raised on a mound of earth, as in traditional rock gardens, and slopes down to the foreground.

What it is used for   Zen gardens are used in the pursuit of self-enlightenment, knowing yourself inside out, through contemplation and meditation. For other benefits, see Meditation and Zen Therapy.

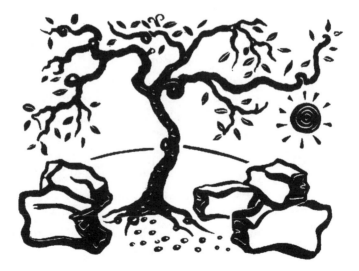

What doctors think

Doctors are happy to agree that sitting in harmonious surroundings does do good. They warn, however, that Zen meditation and its teachings sometimes attract westerners who are alienated from their own culture and families, and may suffer from emotional and mental vulnerability or serious mental breakdown. The general feeling is that you need to be of sound mind to adopt spiritual disciplines, such as meditation, and if such practices are used by the vulnerable or mentally disturbed instead of psychotherapy, there may be an onset or recurrence of mental disturbance.

ZEN THERAPY

Origins

Zen, a form of Buddhism that actually originated in India in the sixth century B.C., came to Japan in the twelfth century and is widely practiced there today.

What it is

Zen is a system of spiritual disciplines and practices, based on Buddhist beliefs and religious practices. It consists of *Za-zen* (sitting meditation), which is practiced every day, sitting cross-legged on cushions, with spine erect, head balanced, alone or in a group; *Sesshin*, or prolonged periods of meditation that may continue for hours or days; and Zen anecdotes, conundrums, and parables, which are renowned for exposing habitual ways of using the mind and encouraging enlightenment and new ways of thinking.

One parable concerns two monks who meet a woman by a flooded river. The young monk backs off, convinced that, as a celibate, he cannot help her because to do so would mean touching her; the older monk, his teacher, picks her up, carries her across, and sets her down on the far bank. Later, the young monk, still upset with his master, asks: "Master, how could you touch that woman?" The master replies: "I set her down at the river bank two hours ago. Are *you* still carrying her?"

What it is used for

The ultimate goal of Zen is self-enlightenment: reaching a state of liberation from the ephemeral and transitory, and attaining the spiritual eternal.

Living in the present moment, the *now,* is considered all essential in Zen. You should be undisturbed by what has happened in the past or what may happen in the future. Various disciplines are used to help an individual stay centered in the present moment. They are also used to help the person release passing materialistic and sexual desires, distractions, and everyday concerns, and to help him or her to detach from ego concerns.

Disciplines are used to increase personal insight and self-awareness, hopefully resulting in enlightenment, the end result of self-discovery: knowing what is real and what is illusory, what will free one from limitations and enable one to reach one's full, mental, emotional, and spiritual potential for the benefit of everyone.

Students of Zen are given their own teacher, who guides them into deeper self-awareness and keeps them on the road to realizing their full potential as a human being. For other benefits, see Meditation.

What doctors think

Doctors emphasize that Zen should not be confused with psychotherapy and warn that there have been instances of the wrong people being attracted to the practice of Zen for the wrong reasons.

Warning

Because the discipline involves much self-confrontation—watching the rising and falling of thought processes, and movements of the mind, feelings, and desires—Zen is considered suitable only for people of sound mind. It is correspondingly considered totally unsuitable for people who have a history of vulnerability; of alienation from their own culture, family, and surroundings; or a history of emotional and mental disturbance that has required medical treatment. The adoption of demanding spiritual disciplines by such people may result in an onset or recurrence of mental disturbance or illness.

ZONE THERAPY

See also Reflexology

Origins

William H. Fitzgerald, an American ear, nose, and throat specialist, developed zone therapy, which subsequently was applied only to the feet and became the field of reflexology.

What it is   Zone therapy is a pressure-point massage therapy that concentrates on ten zones, otherwise known as energy channels, of the body. The practitioner uses the hands or special instruments to apply pressure-point massage to zones that run from the toes to the head, then down to the fingers.

PART TWO

A–Z of Common Conditions and Suitable Complementary Therapies

Several complementary therapies are claimed to be helpful for both preventing and treating individual conditions and disorders; some complementary treatments are more suitable for prevention than for cure. Some of the treatments complement each other; some do not. The practitioner of your chosen therapy or therapies will advise you. It is essential to discuss any alternative treatment you are considering with your doctor. If you do decide to try more than one complementary therapy, mention this to each practitioner.

Choice of treatment is often a matter of personal preference, convenience of access, recommendation, or simply realizing that a particular therapy has worked wonders for somebody you know.

It is important to appreciate that some of the complementary treatments listed under the individual ailments and diseases are more suitable for prevention than for cure. For example, Ayurvedic practitioners claim Ayurveda will benefit everybody, including those who are not ill.*

Whatever therapy you choose, share your anxieties and thoughts with your doctor and complementary therapist—and share any satisfaction with the result, too!

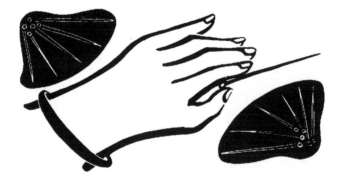

*   As Ayurveda is used for all common ailments and disorders, it has not been listed under every A–Z entry.

ACID STOMACH

This term is used to describe the burning sensation present in some digestive problems and stomach disorders. The symptom is due to an excess of hydrochloric acid in the gastric juice and in the occasional regurgitation of the gastric juice.

Treatment
Acupuncture; biochemic tissue salts therapy; herbal medicine; homeopathy; naturopathy; yoga.

ACNE

A skin condition that primarily affects people between the ages of twelve and twenty-five. Found especially on the face and neck, the condition is characterized by blackheads and pimples.

Treatment
Bach flower remedies; biochemic tissue salts therapy; diet therapy (healthy living); herbal medicine; homeopathy; hydrotherapy; naturopathy; physiotherapy.

ADENOIDS

See Tonsillitis and Adenitis

ADDICTION

The habitual and seemingly uncontrollable dependence on harmful substances, such as alcohol and drugs. It is also used to describe cravings for food, glue sniffing, and cigarettes.

Treatment
Acupuncture; auricular therapy; autogenic training therapy; autosuggestion therapy; behavioral therapy; counseling; dance therapy; flotation therapy; herbal medicine; homeopathy; hydrotherapy; hypnotherapy; megavitamin therapy; naturopathy; psychotherapy; yoga.

AGORAPHOBIA

A neurosis that expresses itself in a fear of open spaces. The fear may be so intense that the sufferer is unable to leave the house.

Treatment
Acupuncture; aromatherapy;
Bach flower remedies;
behavioral therapy; biochemic
tissue salts therapy; herbal
medicine; homeopathy;
psychotherapy; reflexology.

ALCOHOLISM

*A dependence on alcohol, which
can take two forms: episodic
(occasional bouts of heavy
drinking) and persistent (a
steadily increasing inability to
abstain, until the person is
literally living for the next drink).
Alcoholism may eventually render
the person unable to maintain
relationships or go to work, and
result in life-threatening physical,
emotional, and mental-health
problems.*

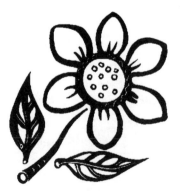

Treatment
Abstinence from alcohol;
auricular therapy; Bach flower
remedies; dance therapy;
flotation therapy; herbal
medicine; hypnotherapy;
megavitamin therapy;
naturopathy; yoga.

ALLERGIES

*A distressing hypersensitivity to
some substance—for example,
dust, food, or pollen. Tiny doses
of the substance can produce a
violent reaction, such as breathing
difficulties in asthmatics and
intense watering of eyes and nose
in hay fever sufferers.*

Treatment
Acupuncture; autosuggestion
therapy; Bach flower
remedies; biofeedback
therapy; homeopathy;
hypnotherapy; kinesiology.

ALOPECIA

See Baldness

AMNESIA

A complete loss of memory of past and/or present events. Some people may experience a gradual deterioration of memory as they age.

Treatment
Bach flower remedies; hypnotherapy.

ANEMIA

A deficiency in the quality or quantity of red corpuscles in the blood that has a host of symptoms, including breathlessness, giddiness, headaches, pallor, and tiredness.

Treatment
Aromatherapy; diet therapy; herbal medicine; homeopathy; hydrotherapy; megavitamin therapy; naturopathy; physiotherapy.

ANAL PROBLEMS

See also Hemorrhoids (Piles), Worms

Fissure is an extremely painful crack or ulcer in the mucous membrane of the anus, commonly caused by constipation. Fistula is an abnormal passage that connects the cavity of one organ with another, or to the surface of the body. It is most likely to occur as the result of an abscess forming after surgery.

Treatment
Aromatherapy; herbal medicine; hydrotherapy.

ANOREXIA

This eating disorder is more common in girls and women, but can affect boys and men. Anorexia is a loss of appetite; anorexia nervosa, often called the "dieter's disease," is a dangerous psychological disorder, a neurosis that can result in a person starving himself or herself to death. Consult your doctor.

Treatment
Acupuncture; art therapy; counseling; dance therapy; hypnotherapy; naturopathy; psychotherapy.

ANXIETY

Anxiety states are triggered and maintained by persistent fears and worries that have no obvious cause but seldom respond to reassurance. If extreme, the person may become unable to cope with the normal everyday stresses of life and relationships. Symptoms commonly include loss of appetite, breathlessness, pain, palpitations, and sleeplessness.

Treatment
Acupuncture; Alexander technique; aromatherapy; auricular therapy; autogenic training therapy; autosuggestion therapy; Bach flower remedies; behavioral therapy; biochemic tissue salts therapy; biofeedback therapy; counseling; dance therapy; flotation therapy; Gestalt therapy; herbal medicine; homeopathy; hydrotherapy; hypnotherapy; massage; meditation; naturopathy; psychotherapy; Rogerian therapy: sound therapy; Tai Chi Ch'uan therapy; yoga.

ARTERIES, HARDENING OF THE

Arteriosclerosis, the hardening and thickening of the arteries, makes the arteries narrow, brittle, and rough, which increases the danger of blood clots. Prevention is the best cure, including avoiding excessive animal fat and carbohydrates, getting regular exercise, and reducing emotional and mental stress. Consult your doctor.

Treatment
Breathing for relaxation therapy; counseling; diet therapy; herbal medicine; naturopathy; psychotherapy.

ARTHRITIS

Arthritis, meaning inflammation of a joint or joints, is really three common diseases: rheumatoid arthritis, osteoarthritis, and gout. Consult your doctor.

Treatment
Acupressure; acupuncture; aromatherapy; auricular therapy; biochemic tissue salts

therapy; chiropractic; cymatic therapy; dance therapy; diet therapy (Hay, macrobiotic); herbal medicine; homeopathy; hydrotherapy; hypnotherapy; massage; naturopathy; osteopathy; physiotherapy; psychotherapy; reflexology; Shiatsu; sound therapy; Tai Chi Ch'uan therapy; yoga.

ASTHMA

Asthma, attacks of breathlessness accompanied by wheezing, are often triggered by allergic reactions or emotional upsets. The difficulty, because of a spasm in the bronchi, is getting the breath out, rather than in. Attacks are distressing and frightening, and severe attacks can be life threatening. Consult your doctor.

Treatment
Acupuncture; Alexander technique; aromatherapy; auricular therapy; autosuggestion therapy; Bach flower remedies; biochemic tissue salts therapy; bioenergetics; biofeedback therapy; chiropractic; diet

therapy; herbal medicine; homeopathy; hydrotherapy; massage; meditation; naturopathy; osteopathy; physiotherapy; reflexology; visualization therapy; yoga.

ATHLETE'S FOOT

A common and contagious fungal infection between the toes, which can be very itchy and uncomfortable, athlete's foot is common among people who regularly go swimming or use communal bathrooms and showers.

Treatment
Aromatherapy; herbal medicine; naturopathy; physiotherapy; reflexology.

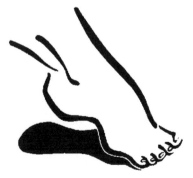

AUTISM

See Special Needs section, page 219

BACK PAIN

Backache and back pain are said to result in more days lost at work than any other condition. A symptom rather than a disease in itself, back pain is often experienced in the lower lumbar region, and it is particularly common in middle-age, overweight men and women, and after pregnancy and childbirth. It can be incapacitating, rendering a person unable to straighten up or move. Consult your doctor.

Treatment
Acupressure; acupuncture; Alexander technique; autogenic training therapy; chiropractic; cymatic therapy; diet therapy; electrotherapy; hydrotherapy; hypnotherapy; kinesiology; massage; osteopathy; physiotherapy; reflexology, Shiatsu; sound therapy; Tai Chi Ch'uan therapy; yoga.

BAD BREATH

Bad breath causes much distress for both the person concerned and others. It may be a warning of deteriorating or existing poor health, and it often accompanies emotional and psychological disturbance.

Treatment
Diet therapy; herbal medicine; homeopathy.

BALDNESS (ALOPECIA)

Some men are very sensitive—almost neurotic—about baldness because they perceive it as a reflection of declining attractiveness, physical energy, and sexual prowess. It is usually even more distressing when it happens to women. It is sometimes a side effect of modern drug treatments, such as chemotherapy, which can in itself cause distress.

Treatment
Diet therapy; homeopathy.

BEDWETTING

Children are usually dry at night by the time they are about three years old, but some suffer from what is known as nocturnal enuresis, uncontrollable loss of urine, and others may revert to bedwetting. Reversion to bedwetting is often the result of insecurity—jealousy of a new-born sibling, a school phobia—making the child want to be a "protected" baby again. Consult your doctor who, having ruled out physical causes such as a urinary tract infection, may recommend a child-guidance clinic.

Treatment
Behavioral therapy; counseling; herbal medicine; hydrotherapy (especially sitz baths); hypnotherapy; psychotherapy.

BEE STINGS

The localized swelling of a bee sting can be dangerous and cause serious breathing difficulties if a person is stung in the mouth or throat or has been sensitized or is allergic to bee stings. If so, call your doctor or emergency service immediately.

Treatment
Bach flower remedies (the rescue remedy); herbal medicine; homeopathy; naturopathy.

For immediate pain relief, extract the bee stinger and treat with ice-cold water into which you have placed some bicarbonate of soda.

BITES, ANIMAL

With animal bites, the possibility of rabies must be considered. Consult a doctor immediately.

Treatment
Bach flower remedies (the rescue remedy); homeopathy; naturopathy.

Clean the bite with the homeopathic remedy: pure tincture of hypericum in cold, boiled water; give Apis as needed for pain.

BLADDER PROBLEMS

The most common bladder problems are bacterial infections, cystitis, kidney stones, and stress incontinence following surgical procedures. Symptoms often include an increased need to urinate and discomfort or pain. Consult your doctor.

Treatment
Aromatherapy; biochemic tissue salts therapy; diet therapy; herbal medicine; homeopathy; hydrotherapy; reflexology.

BLISTERS

A blister is a raised area of the skin that is filled with fluid. It is usually caused by friction—for example, from tight socks and shoes—or trapped heat—for example, from using a tool. To avoid infection, blisters are best left unbroken; if they break, clean the area gently; treat them, for example, with aromatherapy's diluted lavender oil; and cover with a loose bandage.

Treatment
Aromatherapy; biochemic tissue salts therapy; herbal medicine; homeopathy; naturopathy.

BLOOD PRESSURE

Problems arise when the pressure at which the heart pumps blood into the main arteries is too low or too high. Low blood pressure may result from prolonged poor health or a sudden shock; high blood pressure may result from emotional or psychological disturbance, exertion, or stress. Consult your doctor.

Treatment
Low blood pressure:
Acupuncture; aromatherapy; diet therapy (vegetarianism); herbal medicine.

High blood pressure:
Acupuncture; Alexander

technique; aromatherapy;
biofeedback therapy; diet
therapy (Hay); homeopathy;
hydrotherapy; meditation;
naturopathy; reflexology; yoga.

BOILS

*Painful, inflamed abscesses
situated around a hair follicle,
boils that occur on a regular basis
may indicate, for example, poor
diet, poor skin hygiene, poor
health, and the presence of an
actual disease. Consult your
doctor if the problem persists.*

Treatment
Biochemic tissue salts therapy;
diet therapy (healthy living);
herbal medicine; homeopathy;
naturopathy; physiotherapy.

BONE FRACTURES

*In addition to orthodox medical
treatment, including a visit to a
hospital emergency room, the
following complementary therapies
are recommended for bone
fractures.*

Treatment
Cymatic therapy; herbal
medicine; hydrotherapy.

BREAST PROBLEMS

*Breast problems include
inflammatory conditions
associated with breast milk and
breastfeeding. Infection can enter
the breast through a cracked, sore
nipple causing acute
inflammation (mastitis) or breast
abscesses. Consult your family
doctor. The La Leche League has
information pamphlets and local
branches that can support nursing
mothers.*
*Lumps in the breast need to be
seen immediately by your doctor.
Many tumors are benign (not
cancerous), but some may be
cancerous and should be treated
as soon as possible.*

Treatment
Homeopathy.

BRONCHITIS

*This condition, which is common
in both children and adults, is an*

inflammation of the bronchi, the
two branches into which the
windpipe divides before entering
the lungs. It often begins with a
common cold or cough or a bout
of influenza. Consult your doctor.

Treatment
Acupuncture; aromatherapy;
autogenic training therapy;
biochemic tissue salts therapy;
breathing for relaxation
therapy; herbal medicine;
homeopathy; hydrotherapy;
meditation; naturopathy;
physiotherapy; reflexology;
yoga.

BRUISES

Bruises are usually superficial
tissue injuries. The discoloration
that results from damage to the
tissue and underlying blood
vessels can be a dramatic, dark
purplish-blue fading to various
shades of brown, green, and
yellow before disappearing
altogether. Consult your doctor if
there is a possibility of any serious
injury having been caused by the
impact.

Treatment
Aromatherapy; Bach flower
remedies (the rescue remedy);
herbal medicine; homeopathy;
hydrotherapy; naturopathy.

BULIMIA

This eating disorder, which
consists of eating to
excess—bingeing on food until
vomiting becomes
inevitable—often accompanies
anorexia nervosa (see page 153).
Like anorexia nervosa, bulimia is
thought to be on the increase,
especially in women between
puberty and twenty-five years of
age. Although it has dramatic
physical effects, it is a
psychological disorder, a neurosis
that can have life-threatening
consequences.

Treatment
Art therapy; Bach flower
remedies; counseling; dance
therapy; hypnotherapy;
naturopathy; psychotherapy.

BUNIONS

A disfiguring swelling, bunions are usually found over the joint of a big toe and may or may not be painful. They are usually caused by wearing shoes, socks, or stockings that are too tight.

Treatment
Acupuncture; aromatherapy; herbal medicine; naturopathy.

BURNS AND SCALDS

The seriousness of burns and scalds ranges from first-degree burns (no tissue destruction) to sixth-degree burns (the charring of a whole limb). According to the degree, burns and scalds may be treated by first-aid procedures, or they may need the urgent attention of a hospital emergency room or burns unit.

Treatment
Aromatherapy; Bach flower remedies (the rescue remedy); and homeopathy can be used to promote recovery from burn surgery or other medical treatment.

For superficial burns, try the homeopathic remedy of ten drops of hypericum lotion to a glass of water applied to the affected area, followed by taking a few drops of Bach rescue remedy in water for shock.

BURSITIS

This condition, sometimes referred to as "housemaid's knee," "miner's elbow," and "tennis elbow," is an inflammation of the bursa, the fluid-filled cavities between tendons and bones. Bursitis may be a repetitive stress injury caused by overuse.

Treatment
Aromatherapy; herbal medicine; homeopathy; hydrotherapy; massage; naturopathy; physiotherapy.

CANDIDA

See Thrush

CATARACTS

A cataract is a clouding of the lens of the eye, which can lead to blindness. Consult your doctor, who will refer you to an eye specialist.

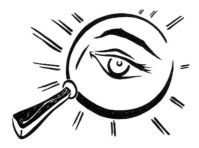

Treatment
Naturopaths claim that they, too, can offer help. Nutritionists with ophthalmic training may help delay the onset of cataracts, if consulted early enough.

CATARRH

Catarrh is inflammation of the mucous membrane. There is usually no sign of inflammation, but plenty of evidence of mucous discharge.

Treatment
Acupressure; acupuncture; aromatherapy; biochemic tissue salts therapy; herbal medicine; homeopathy; hydrotherapy; kinesiology; massage; naturopathy; physiotherapy; reflexology.

CELIAC DISEASE

Sufferers of celiac disease are deficient in an enzyme needed to digest gluten. Once a gluten-free diet is started, recovery should be swift.

Treatment
Diet therapy (nutritional); herbal medicine; nutrition; physiotherapy.

CHAPPED SKIN

Inflamed, flaky patches of skin, sometimes accompanied by painful cracks, usually results from overexposure to cold, rain, or wind, and mainly affects the face, hands, and legs.

Treatment
Aromatherapy; herbal remedies; homeopathy; naturopathy.

CHICKEN POX

A common, usually mild, but very infectious childhood ailment, chicken pox is much better endured in childhood than in adulthood, when the symptoms are usually much more severe. A pinkish rash may precede crops of small blisters on the abdomen, back, chest, face, scalp, and limbs. The blisters become pustular, then dry out and form scabs. Scarring may result if the scabs are scratched.

Treatment
Aromatherapy; biochemic tissue salts therapy; herbal medicine; homeopathy; hydrotherapy; naturopathy.

CHILBLAINS

An itchy, localized, inflammatory condition of the skin, chilblains usually occur as a reaction to cold on exposed parts of the hands and feet.

Treatment
Diet therapy (nutritional); herbal medicine; homeopathy; massage; naturopathy.

CHILDHOOD INFECTIONS

See the individual conditions

CHRONIC FATIGUE SYNDROME (CFS)

Also called chronic fatigue immune dysfunction syndrome (CFIDS), this illness is characterized by fatigue, malaise, and feeling unable to cope with the ordinary stresses of life and relationships. Other symptoms include dizziness, headaches, nausea, constant tiredness, marked muscular weakness, cognitive difficulties, and a perceived loss of control of the sympathetic nervous system. Consult your doctor.

Treatment
Acupuncture; Alexander technique; aromatherapy; autogenic training therapy; autosuggestion therapy; Bach flower remedies; counseling; diet therapy; herbal medicine; homeopathy; hydrotherapy; hypnotherapy; massage; megavitamin therapy; naturopathy; psychotherapy.

CIRCULATION PROBLEMS

For problems with circulation, consult your doctor.

Treatment
Aromatherapy; biochemic tissue salts therapy; electrotherapy; herbal medicine; hydrotherapy; massage; meditation; naturopathy; Tai Chi Ch'uan therapy.

CLAUSTROPHOBIA

An uncontrollable fear of being in confined places, claustrophobia may cause a confined person to

panic, hyperventilate (overbreathe), and even thrash around and become violent.

Treatment
Acupressure; Bach flower remedies; behavioral therapy; breathing for relaxation therapy; counseling; homeopathy; hypnotherapy; psychotherapy; reflexology.

COLD SORES (HERPES)

An infectious eruption caused by a virus, cold sores usually appear around the mouth.

Treatment
Biochemic tissue salts therapy; diet therapy; homeopathy; naturopathy; physiotherapy.

COLDS

The common cold, usually caused by a virus, can have very unpleasant symptoms.

Treatment
Acupressure; aromatherapy;

biochemic tissue salts therapy;
herbal medicine; homeopathy;
kinesiology; naturopathy.

COLIC

*Colic is characterized by gripping,
spasmodic pain, usually in the
intestine. The pain may vary from
slight to intolerable. Consult your
doctor.*

Treatment
Aromatherapy; herbal
medicine.

COLITIS

*Inflammation of the colon,
accompanied by discomfort in the
lower abdomen and punctuated by
sharp pains, colitis can be caused
by bacterial infection or food
poisoning. Chronic colitis is
usually caused by constipation or
overuse of laxatives. The chronic
version usually occurs in people
of anxious disposition, and
psychological treatment may be
necessary. First consult your doctor.*

Treatment
Acupressure; acupuncture;
Alexander technique;
autogenic training therapy;
counseling; diet therapy;
herbal medicine; homeopathy;
hydrotherapy; hypnotherapy;
naturopathy; psychotherapy.

COMPULSIVE
BEHAVIOR

See Obsessive-Compulsive
Behavior

CONJUNCTIVITIS

*Inflammation of the conjunctiva,
the membrane that covers the
front of the eye, is experienced as
"stickiness" of the eyelid, grit
beneath the eyelid, and pain and
excessive watering of the eye.
Consult your doctor if symptoms
persist longer than two days.*

Treatment
Herbal medicine;
homeopathy; naturopathy.

CONSTIPATION

Difficulty or infrequency of bowel movements may be the result of a poor diet; of bad bowel habits, such as the habitual ignoring of the initial impulse to evacuate the bowel; of bowel obstruction; or of stress.

Treatment
Diet therapy; herbal medicine; homeopathy; hydrotherapy; naturopathy; physiotherapy; reflexology.

CORNS

A thickened area of skin, usually on the toes, corns are caused by the friction of too-tight shoes, socks, or stockings. They can be painful, so prevention is certainly desirable.

Treatment
Herbal medicine; naturopathy.

COUGHS

A symptom of many disorders of the lungs, including infections such as bronchitis, a cough may be irritating, dry, and accompanied by phlegm. Contact your doctor to rule out life-threatening conditions.

Treatment
Acupuncture; aromatherapy; biochemic tissue salts therapy; herbal medicine; homeopathy; naturopathy; physiotherapy.

CRAMPS

A very painful muscle spasm, a cramp may be triggered by sitting or lying in a way that puts pressure on a nerve—this is the agonizing leg cramp you wake up with in bed. Swimmer's cramp is thought to be caused by cold, and a third kind of cramp is thought to be caused by excessive loss of potassium salt. Although unpleasant at first, rubbing the muscle usually eases the pain and brings a bout to a quick end. The muscles may continue to feel "bunched" and uncomfortable for some time.

Treatment
Aromatherapy; autogenic training therapy; biochemic tissue salts therapy; herbal medicine; homeopathy; hydrotherapy; massage; osteopathy; naturopathy.

CROUP

A distressing cough caused by inflammation or spasm of the larynx, croup affects babies and children and makes it difficult for them to breathe. Consult your doctor.

Treatment
Aromatherapy; herbal medicine; hydrotherapy; naturopathy.

CYSTITIS

Inflammation of the bladder or the urethra caused by an infection, cystitis is experienced as a burning sensation when urinating and an intense desire to pass urine immediately after urinating. The urine may be cloudy and have a strong odor. Consult your doctor, as a persistent bladder infection can spread to the kidneys.

Treatment
Aromatherapy; biochemic tissue salts therapy; diet therapy; herbal medicine; homeopathy; hydrotherapy; naturopathy; reflexology.

DANDRUFF

Dandruff is a flaky, scaly skin that can occur on the eyebrows and scalp.

Treatment
Aromatherapy; diet therapy; herbal medicine; naturopathy; physiotherapy.

DEPRESSION

See also Manic-Depressive Illness

Depression may be characterized by a feeling of hopelessness; a conviction that nothing is worthwhile; a reluctance to be with others, to get up, or to go out; little or no interest in anything; and a constant urge to cry. Consider consulting a doctor or psychotherapist if depression is accompanied by thoughts of suicide.

Treatment
Acupuncture; Alexander technique; aromatherapy; autogenic training therapy; autosuggestion therapy; Bach flower remedies; counseling; dance therapy; diet therapy; herbal medicine; homeopathy; hydrotherapy; hypnotherapy; kinesiology; massage; megavitamin therapy.

DIABETES

Diabetes, which results from an inadequate production of insulin, or by insulin insensitivity of the cells, other glandular organs, and body tissues, is characterized by a reduced or nonexistent ability to metabolize carbohydrates. Consult your doctor. In addition to medical advice, the following may be helpful.

Treatment
Diet therapy; naturopathy; physiotherapy; yoga.

DIARRHEA

Frequent evacuation of the bowels, diarrhea may be caused by diet, bacterial infection, or food poisoning. This condition may indicate serious illness and can be life threatening for a baby;. Consult your doctor.

Treatment
Aromatherapy; diet therapy; herbal medicine; homeopathy; naturopathy; Shiatsu.

DIGESTIVE DISORDERS

Discomfort or pain caused by intestinal gas, digestive disorders may be accompanied by headache, nausea, and vomiting.

Treatment
Acupressure; acupuncture; aromatherapy; auricular therapy; autogenic training therapy; ayurvedic medicine; biochemic tissue salts therapy; breathing for relaxation therapy; diet therapy (Hay, macrobiotic); herbal medicine; kinesiology; naturopathy; reflexology; Shiatsu.

DIZZINESS

Dizziness may include giddiness, or a sense of spinning, losing one's balance, or falling. If it occurs frequently, consult your doctor.

Treatment
Acupressure; chiropractic; naturopathy.

DUODENAL ULCERS

See Ulcers

DYSENTERY

An acute infection of the large intestine, dysentery may be

accompanied by abdominal pain, diarrhea, and blood and mucous in the feces. Consult your doctor.

Treatment
Naturopathy.

EARACHES

Earaches may indicate congestion, inflammation, or infection of the external or middle ear. The symptoms may include discharge, fever, pain, and throbbing. Serious ear infections can cause hearing damage in young children, so consulting a doctor is recommended.

Treatment
Diet therapy; herbal medicine; homeopathy; physiotherapy.

ECZEMA

An inflamed reddening, and sometimes blistering, of the skin, eczema can occur on any part of the body.

Treatment
Acupuncture; aromatherapy; autogenic training therapy;

ayurvedic medicine; Bach flower remedies; herbal medicine; homeopathy; naturopathy; reflexology.

EDEMA

See Fluid Retention (Edema)

EMPHYSEMA

Emphysema is a degenerative disease of the lungs that causes breathlessness, coughing, expectoration (coughing up of phlegm), and wheezing.

Treatment
Acupuncture; aromatherapy; diet therapy; herbal medicine; naturopathy; physiotherapy.

EPILEPSY

Epilepsy is characterized by sudden loss of consciousness, perhaps with some jerking of the extremities; seizures may be short (petit mal) or severe (grand mal).

Treatment
Aromatherapy; Bach flower remedies; diet therapy; naturopathy; physiotherapy. Control the immediate environment to eliminate flickering lights or sensations, as this can trigger a seizure.

EYESTRAIN

Eyestrain may occur at any age. Symptoms of eyestrain include frequent blinking, rubbing of the eyes, redness, and headache.

Treatment
Acupressure; herbal medicine; homeopathy; naturopathy. Use protection in bright sunlight, and always have well-positioned, adequate lighting when studying or doing any kind of close work. It is essential to have eyes checked regularly by an optometrist.

FAINTING

A distressing temporary loss of consciousness, fainting is caused

by a deficiency of the blood supply
to the brain. It is usually
preceded by dizziness and can
sometimes be prevented by
lowering the head between the
knees. If it is a frequent
occurrence, contact your doctor.

Treatment
Acupressure; Bach flower
remedies; homeopathy.

FATIGUE (EXHAUSTION)

*A complete lack of energy and
tiredness, fatigue may be
accompanied by feelings of
depression, lethargy, weakness,
and a lack of desire to do
anything. The cause of continual
fatigue or tiredness should be
investigated and addressed. It
may be physical, emotional, or
psychological. Consult your doctor
if exhaustion is prolonged.*

Treatment
Acupressure; acupuncture;
Alexander technique;
aromatherapy; breathing and
relaxation therapy; diet
therapy; herbal medicine;

homeopathy; hydrotherapy;
kinesiology; massage;
physiotherapy.

FEAR

*This unpleasant emotion is caused
by the anticipation of danger. If
fear is experienced in the absence
of danger, complementary
remedies may help alleviate it.*

Treatment
Bach flower remedies;
behavioral therapy;
counseling; herbal medicine;
hypnotherapy; meditation;
naturopathy; psychotherapy.

FEVER

*An above-normal
temperature—normal is
considered to be 98.6° F (37°
C)—fever may be accompanied by
lethargy and hot, dry or wet skin.*

Treatment
Biochemic tissue salts therapy;
herbal medicine; homeopathy;
hydrotherapy; naturopathy;
physiotherapy (if advised).

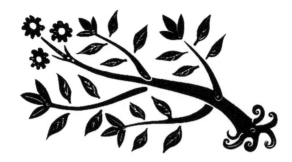

FIBROSIS

*A term used to describe a sudden
onset of pain and stiffness, fibrosis
is thought to arise from injury or
strain to ligaments. It may be
accompanied by muscle spasm.*

Treatment
Massage; osteopathy; sound
therapy.

FLATULENCE

*Excessive intestinal gas, sometimes
accompanied by intestinal
discomfort, flatulence is usually
caused by swallowing too much
air while eating or drinking; it
can also be caused by anxiety.*

Treatment
Aromatherapy; diet therapy;
herbal medicine; homeopathy;
hypnotherapy; naturopathy;
physiotherapy.

A half teaspoon of
bicarbonate of soda in warm
water usually relieves the
immediate symptoms.

FLUID RETENTION (EDEMA)

*An abnormal buildup of watery
fluid in body tissues and cavities,
fluid retention is most commonly
seen as swelling of the ankles. As
fluid retention can be an
indication of heart disease or
renal disorder, it is important to
consult your family doctor.*

Treatment
Acupuncture; herbal medicine;
massage; naturopathy.

FOOD POISONING

Caused by eating bacteria-contaminated food, this acute illness is accompanied by pain in the abdomen, diarrhea, and vomiting. For anything but mild attacks, consult your family doctor.

Treatment
Herbal medicine; homeopathy; hydrotherapy; naturopathy.

FOOT PROBLEMS

See also Athlete's Foot, Bunions, Corns

Problems of the feet are often associated with the wearing of tight or improper footwear.

Treatment
Aromatherapy; hydrotherapy; massage; osteopathy; reflexology.

FROZEN SHOULDER

See also Bursitis

"Frozen shoulder" refers to a particular type of bursitis and is an inflammation of the bursa in the shoulder, accompanied by pain and stiffness.

Treatment
Acupressure; aromatherapy; autogenic training therapy; chiropractic; herbal medicine; homeopathy.

FUNGAL INFECTIONS

See Athlete's Foot, Thrush

GALLSTONES

Stones in the gall bladder are of three varieties: cholesterol stones (usually a single stone), pigment stones (usually multiple stones), and mixed stones. Gallstones may exist for years without pain, then suddenly cause intense pain accompanied by high fever, rigor, and vomiting.

Treatment
Acupuncture; diet therapy; herbal medicine; home-

opathy; hydrotherapy;
naturopathy.

GAS

See Flatulence

GASTRIC ULCERS

See Ulcers

GLANDULAR FEVER

An acute infection, glandular fever may be accompanied by fever, sore throat, swelling of cervical and other lymph glands, and enlargement of the spleen. Consult your doctor.

Treatment
Biochemic tissue salts therapy; herbal medicine; homeopathy; naturopathy. Counseling and hypnotherapy can help with the associated depression.

GOUT

Gout is a metabolic disease characterized by sudden, acute

inflammation of a joint with pain, tenderness, and swelling, often involving the first joint at the base of the big toe. It is due to the buildup of uric salt acids.

Treatment
Acupressure; acupuncture; aromatherapy; auricular therapy; biochemic tissue salts therapy; cymatic therapy; diet therapy; herbal medicine; homeopathy; hydrotherapy; hypnotherapy; massage; naturopathy; osteopathy; physiotherapy; psychotherapy; reflexology; sound therapy; Tai Chi Ch'uan therapy; yoga.

HANGOVER

The extremely unpleasant side effects of overindulgence in alcohol, a hangover may include headache, giddiness, nausea, and a feeling of disorientation.

Treatment
Herbal medicine; homeopathy; hydrotherapy; naturopathy.

HAY FEVER

Hay fever, an allergic response to pollen, can be triggered by other allergens. It consists of a profuse, watery nasal discharge, sneezing, and watery eyes, and may be accompanied by asthmatic-type symptoms.

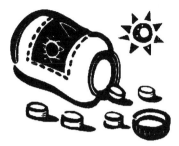

Treatment

Acupuncture; auricular therapy; biochemic tissue salts therapy; homeopathy; hypnotherapy; naturopathy.

HEADACHES

See also Migraines

Consisting of pain in or around the head, headaches differ from migraines, which are recurrent headaches confined to one side of the head or eye and often accompanied by visual disturbances, nausea, or vomiting.

Treatment

Acupuncture; Alexander technique; aromatherapy; behavioral therapy; biofeedback; bioenergetics; chiropractic; diet therapy; herbal medicine; homeopathy; hydrotherapy; kinesiology; massage; naturopathy; osteopathy, Shiatsu.

HEARTBURN

See Digestive Disorders

HEART DISEASE

Consult your doctor for any sign of heart disease; she or he may refer you to a heart specialist.

Treatment

Diet therapy (vegetarian); breathing for relaxation therapy; hydrotherapy (avoid the sudden shock of hot and cold); homeopathy; meditation; physiotherapy; yoga.

HEAT RASH

Also called prickly heat rash, this is a localized or generalized pinkish rash, which may include small, watery, red pimples and blisters. Heat rash is due to blockage of the sweat glands caused by excessive perspiration, and may be aggravated by wearing too many clothes, especially clothes made from synthetic fibers instead of cotton, linen, or silk, or becoming overheated for prolonged periods. It is also referred to as prickly heat.

Treatment
Herbal medicine; hydrotherapy (to cool down); naturopathy.

HEMORRHOIDS (PILES)

Hemorrhoids are internal or external varicose veins of the anal region; the external veins protrude as painful, dilated swellings. Symptoms include burning, itching, and pain when evacuating the bowels.

Treatment
Aromatherapy; autogenic training therapy; herbal medicine; hydrotherapy (especially cold and hot compresses and sitz baths); homeopathy; naturopathy; yoga.

HERPES

See Cold Sores

HICCUPS

Repeated body-shaking spasms, often preceded by drinking or eating too quickly—or laughing too much.

Treatment
Herbal medicine; naturopathy.

HIVES

An allergic reaction to food, hives are often a response to chocolate, strawberries, shellfish or, less commonly, antibiotics or pollen. The reaction results in reddish, itching, circular wheals.

Treatment
Herbal medicine; homeopathy; naturopathy; physiotherapy.
     The best treatment is to identify and avoid the allergen.

HYPERACTIVITY

A behavioral disorder, more common in children than adults, hyperactivity is often accompanied by emotional instability, destructive behavior, an inability to concentrate, and temper tantrums.

Treatment
Behavioral therapy; dance therapy; diet therapy; homeopathy; hydrotherapy (especially saunas); massage; megavitamin therapy; naturopathy.

HYPERGLYCEMIA

An excess of sugar in the blood caused by the pancreas not producing enough insulin, hyperglycemia may be a sign of diabetes. Consult your doctor. The following may be useful to support orthodox treatment.

Treatment
Diet therapy; naturopathy; reflexology.

HYPERTENSION

Hypertension, or high blood pressure, may be accompanied by dizziness, loss of energy, fatigue, insomnia, and nervousness.

Treatment
Breathing for relaxation therapy; diet therapy; hydrotherapy (especially alternate warm and cool showers); meditation; yoga.

HYPERVENTILATION

Excessive breathing due to an abnormal loss of carbon dioxide

*from the blood, hyperventilation
often accompanies anxiety,
hysteria, and panic attacks.*

Treatment
Biofeedback therapy;
breathing for relaxation
therapy; hypnotherapy; yoga.

HYPOGLYCEMIA

*An abnormal decrease in blood
sugar, hypoglycemia may be
accompanied by tiredness,
dizziness, and fainting.*

Treatment
Diet therapy; naturopathy.

HYPOTHERMIA

*A chilling of the body that, if left
unchecked, can lead to permanent
damage and, ultimately, death.
Hypothermia is usually discovered
as an emergency but can happen
in any environment.*

Treatment
Diet therapy; exercise;
massage; naturopathy.

HYSTERIA

*A loss of self-control, hysteria is
characterized by emotional
outbursts, including expressions of
frustration and helplessness to
escape from, perhaps, an
intolerable situation. Hysterical
reactions may appear as disorders
of bodily functions without
physical disease, including
blindness, deafness, dumbness,
tremors, and even paralysis.
Underlying problems need
professional help.*

Treatment
Bach flower remedies;
counseling; hypnotherapy;
psychotherapy.

IMPETIGO

*A very contagious skin infection,
commonly caused by staphylococci
but occasionally by streptococcus,
impetigo is characterized by
blisters that form greenish-yellow
crusts.*

Treatment
Diet therapy; herbal medicine;
naturopathy.

INCONTINENCE, URINARY STRESS

Incontinence is an involuntary dribble of urine that occurs, for example, when coughing, laughing, lifting, running, or sneezing. It is fairly common in women who have given birth to several children or after gynecological surgery. If severe, consider consulting a doctor.

Treatment
Diet therapy; electrotherapy; exercise therapy (especially pelvic); herbal medicine; hydrotherapy (especially hot and cold sitz baths); naturopathy; physiotherapy.

INDIGESTION

See Digestive Disorders

INFERTILITY

See Special Needs section, page 223

INFLUENZA

An infectious disease caused by a virus, influenza symptoms include fever, headache, back and limb aches, common cold symptoms, and inflammatory complications in the respiratory organs.

Treatment
Biochemic tissue salts therapy; herbal medicine; homeopathy; naturopathy.

INSECT BITES AND STINGS

Some people are dangerously allergic to insect bites and stings—especially bee and wasp stings—and need instant medical attention to prevent severe reactions and possibly death. The following recommendations are for people who are not severely allergic to insect stings.

Treatment
Herbal medicine; naturopathy.
    Having removed the stinger, if there is one, apply ice to the area. The homeo-pathic remedy of 25 drops of

Apis tincture in a small amount of water, dabbed onto the bite four to six times a day, is said to help. Traditional remedies include dabbing wasp stings with vinegar, and bee and ant stings with a paste made from water and bicarbonate of soda.

INSOMNIA

See also Sleep Disorders

Short- or long-term difficulty in getting to sleep or staying asleep is often triggered by emotional disturbance, such as bereavement or loss of one's job, but may have a physical cause, such as pain, overeating, or keeping irregular hours. The sufferer may become exhausted, irritable, and depressed.

Treatment
Acupuncture; aromatherapy; autogenic training therapy; behavioral therapy; biofeedback therapy; breathing for relaxation therapy; diet therapy; flotation therapy; herbal medicine; homeopathy; hydrotherapy; hypnotherapy; massage; meditation; physiotherapy; Shiatsu; yoga.

IRRITABLE BOWEL SYNDROME

Irritable bowel syndrome is experienced as muscular spasms and a buildup of pressure within the bowel. Other symptoms may include alternating bouts of constipation and diarrhea, and pain, particularly in the left lower

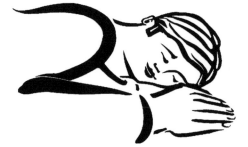

abdomen. *Anxiety, nervousness, and stress may aggravate the condition. Consult your doctor.*

Treatment
Acupressure; acupuncture; Alexander technique; autogenic training therapy; counseling; diet therapy; herbal medicine; homeopathy; hydrotherapy; hypnotherapy; naturopathy; psychotherapy.

ITCHES

The reason for an itch is usually known—for example, the existence of a skin condition, such as eczema, athlete's foot, or chilblains—but general itching may have no obvious cause. Gout, jaundice, allergic reactions to drugs, and other serious conditions may be accompanied by itching. If it continues, consult your doctor.

Treatment
Diet therapy; herbal medicine; naturopathy.

JAUNDICE

Jaundice is a yellowish discoloration of the skin and white of the eye due to the presence of bile pigment in the blood. It can be an indication of a serious disorder, such as cirrhosis, hepatitis, or inflammatory conditions. Consult your doctor.

Treatment
Herbal medicine; homeopathy; reflexology.

JET LAG

Jet lag occurs following long flights and is probably caused by a disruption of the body's circadian rhythms. The symptoms of jet lag, which are rather like those of a hangover, may include headache, giddiness, lethargy, irritability, nausea, and feeling disoriented, dazed, and generally below par.

Treatment
Aromatherapy; autogenic training therapy; herbal medicine; hypnotherapy; massage.

JOINT PROBLEMS

Joint problems may stem from an injury; any inflammatory condition that affects them is termed arthritis. Acute arthritis may be caused by infection or a complication of other diseases, such as rheumatic fever, osteoarthritis (see page 190), and gout (see page 174). Consult your doctor.

Treatment
Acupressure; acupuncture; chiropractic; homeopathy; hydrotherapy; massage; osteopathy; reflexology; Shiatsu.

KIDNEY COMPLAINTS

Consult your doctor for any problem of the kidneys. He or she will most likely refer you to a kidney specialist.

Treatment
Acupressure; acupuncture; homeopathy; naturopathy; reflexology; Tai Chi Ch'uan therapy.

KIDNEY STONES

The formation of gravel or stone in the kidneys gives rise to a dull, dragging pain in the lower back, groin, leg, or testicle, often triggered by motion. A sudden, sharp pain may indicate that a stone has entered the ureter, and this is often accompanied by an increased need to urinate; nausea; vomiting; and agonizing pain. Consult your doctor.

Treatment
Diet therapy; herbal medicine; homeopathy; hydrotherapy (especially sitz baths); naturopathy; physiotherapy.

LARYNGITIS

Inflammation of the larynx and vocal chords is usually due to infection or misuse, such as too much shouting. It leads to hoarseness and sometimes total loss of voice. Laryngitis is often accompanied by fever and a ticklish cough.

Treatment
Acupressure; herbal medicine

(compresses and gargles);
homeopathy; naturopathy.

LEG ULCERS

See Ulcers

LUMBAGO

*Lumbago, a common condition
involving muscular inflammation
of the lumbar region, gives rise to
an ache or pain in the lower
back, buttocks, calf, foot, or thigh,
at times making movement
difficult or even impossible.
Complete rest may be necessary.*

Treatment
Acupressure; acupuncture;
Alexander technique;
autogenic training therapy;
biochemic tissue salts therapy;
chiropractic; cymatic therapy;
diet therapy; electrotherapy;
hydrotherapy; hypnotherapy;
massage; osteopathy;
physiotherapy; reflexology;
sound therapy; Tai Chi
Ch'uan therapy; yoga.

MANIC-DEPRESSIVE ILLNESS

See also Depression

*A mood disorder in which
periods of depression alternate
with periods of excitement, manic-
depressive illness may also involve
delusions and thoughts of or
attempts at suicide. If suicidal
thoughts are occurring, consult a
doctor.*
*Symptoms include a slowing
down of the faculties,
characterized by a loss of
confidence and interest in people
and events. Sleeplessness and a
loss of appetite for both food and
sex are common. The manic
phase is accompanied by
hyperactivity and bizarre behavior.*

Treatment
Biochemic tissue salts therapy;
dance therapy; homeopathy;
psychotherapy.

MEASLES

*A very infectious childhood viral
disease, measles can give rise to
serious complications, such as*

bronchopneumonia. *Symptoms include chest infection, conjunctivitis, and rash. Consult your doctor.*

Treatment
Diet therapy; herbal medicine; homeopathy; hydrotherapy.

MENOPAUSAL PROBLEMS

A natural stage of a woman's life, menopause usually occurs between forty-five and fifty years of age, when hormonal changes eventually result in a cessation of menstruation. Accompanying symptoms can include anxiety attacks, cold sweats, depression, hot flashes, palpitations, irritability, and painful sexual intercourse due to lack of vaginal secretion.

Women who regard menopause as a positive step—a new phase of life, free from biological-clock considerations of menstruation, pregnancy, and childbirth; and a time to allow other aspects of their being to be developed—may suffer fewer symptoms.

Treatment
Acupuncture; aromatherapy; breathing for relaxation therapy; counseling; diet

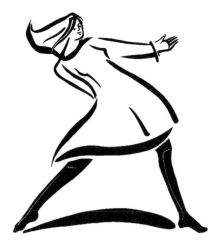

therapy; herbal medicine;
homeopathy; hydrotherapy;
massage; meditation;
naturopathy; physiotherapy;
psychotherapy; yoga.

MENSTRUAL PROBLEMS

See also Premenstrual Tension

*Menstrual problems may include
complete absence of, infrequency
of, difficult or painful, or
bleeding between periods. There
are a host of possible causes for
each condition, and the possibility
of physical disease should be
investigated first. Consult your
doctor.*

Treatment
Acupuncture; Alexander
technique; aromatherapy;
biochemic tissue salts therapy;
breathing for relaxation
therapy; diet therapy; herbal
medicine; homeopathy;
hydrotherapy (for pain relief);
hypnotherapy; naturopathy;
physiotherapy; reflexology.

MIGRAINES

*Migraines resemble headaches but
unlike the generalized pain of
headache, the pain is usually
confined to one side of the head
or eye and may be accompanied
by nausea, vomiting, and acute
sensitivity to light. Consult your
doctor.*

Treatment
Acupressure; acupuncture;
auricular therapy; autogenic
training therapy; biochemic
tissue salts therapy;
bioenergetics; biofeedback
therapy; breathing for
relaxation therapy; diet
therapy; herbal medicine;
homeopathy; hydrotherapy
(especially cold compresses);
hypnotherapy; massage;
reflexology; sound therapy;
yoga.

MINERAL DEFICIENCY

*Mineral deficiency takes its toll
on a person's general well-being
and health. The minerals sodium,
potassium, and magnesium are*

usually present in a reasonable diet; phosphorus, sulfur, calcium, iron, iodine, and zinc are more likely to be lacking in the diet. A well- balanced diet will usually correct the deficiency. Seek dietary advice.

Treatment
Biochemic tissue salts therapy; diet therapy; kinesiology.

MOOD SWINGS

First amiable, then irritable; first smiling, then crying; first decisive, then indecisive. Such mood swings can be a serious problem, affecting the whole of life and making relationships difficult. The underlying cause may be physical, emotional, or psychological. Seek professional help.

Treatment
Acupuncture; Alexander technique; aromatherapy; autogenic training therapy; autosuggestion therapy; Bach flower remedies; counseling; diet therapy; herbal medicine; homeopathy; hydrotherapy;

hypnotherapy; massage; megavitamin therapy; psychotherapy.

MORNING SICKNESS

Morning sickness mainly affects the first three months of pregnancy. When seeking help, always mention that you are pregnant.

Treatment
Herbal medicine; homeopathy; naturopathy.

MOSQUITO BITES

See Insect Bites and Stings

MOTION SICKNESS

Some people are much more susceptible to motion, both irregular and rhythmical, than others. Symptoms of travel sickness are dizziness, nausea and vomiting, headache, pallor, and sweating.

Treatment
Acupressure; acupuncture; aromatherapy; Bach flower remedies; herbal medicine; homeopathy; hypnotherapy; naturopathy.

MUMPS

A contagious childhood disease caused by a virus, mumps is accompanied by fever, painful swelling, especially in front of the ears, and tenderness of the salivary glands, producing the characteristic swollen face. Eating is uncomfortable and painful. Consult your doctor.

Treatment
Biochemic tissue salts therapy; herbal medicine; homeopathy; naturopathy.

MUSCULAR TENSION AND WEAKNESS

Tension and weakness in muscles can arise from several causes, so the condition must first be investigated and a doctor consulted if necessary.

Treatment
Alexander technique; biochemic tissue salts therapy; breathing for relaxation therapy; hydrotherapy; kinesiology; meditation; physiotherapy; yoga.

NAUSEA AND VOMITING

Nausea and vomiting may indicate nothing more serious than an overindulgence in food, drink, or activity; likewise, both may stem from a serious condition that needs urgent medical attention. They are sometimes an early symptom of pregnancy, and can arise from emotional upsets and psychological shock and trauma.

Treatment
Acupressure; biochemic tissue salts therapy; herbal medicine; homeopathy; naturopathy.

For overindulgence, drinking three drops of Olbas oil, diluted in a little water, has been known to work wonders.

NECK PAIN

Neck pain may result from poor posture, muscle stiffness, tension, or injury. Swelling in the neck, usually visible, could be caused by mumps (see page 187), glandular fever (see page 174), or tonsillitis (see page 205). Consult your doctor.

Treatment
Acupuncture; Alexander technique; chiropractic; kinesiology; massage; osteopathy; physiotherapy; reflexology; yoga.

NERVOUS DISORDERS

A general term used to describe a multitude of ills, nervous disorders include anxiety, depression, and physical, emotional, and psychological disturbance that undermine a person's ability to cope with the everyday stresses of life and relationships. The type of professional help needed will be based on the underlying cause.

Treatment
Acupuncture; Alexander technique; aromatherapy; art therapy; auricular therapy; autosuggestion therapy; autogenic training therapy; Bach flower remedies; behavioral therapy; biochemic tissue salts therapy; counseling; dance therapy; diet therapy; herbal medicine; homeopathy; hydrotherapy; hypnotherapy; massage; megavitamin therapy; music therapy; yoga.

NEURALGIA AND NEURITIS

Inflammation or irritation of a nerve, neuralgia and neuritis are associated with burning, tingling, numbness, and localized and generalized pain.

Treatment
Acupressure; acupuncture; aromatherapy; biochemic tissue salts therapy; chiropractic; diet therapy; hydrotherapy; massage; naturopathy; osteopathy; physiotherapy; sound therapy.

NOSE AND THROAT AILMENTS

See Colds, Influenza, Laryngitis, Sinusitis, Tonsillitis and Adenitis

OBESITY

Obese people may be carrying so much weight that both the quality and quantity of life are affected. Effects of obesity may cause serious discomfort, including breathlessness; chafing of fatty parts; damage to lungs, heart, knees, and feet; and many other serious and even life-threatening problems, such as high blood pressure and hardening of the arteries. Being overweight may particularly be a problem for children. Consult your doctor, who will first rule out physiological causes, such as a hormonal imbalance.

Treatment
Acupuncture; breathing for relaxation therapy; chiropractic; dance therapy; diet therapy; homeopathy; hydrotherapy (particularly sauna and hot and cold showers to stimulate circulation); physiotherapy; yoga.

Counseling and psychotherapy may be necessary if the person concerned is deeply upset by his or her obesity.

OBSESSIVE-COMPULSIVE BEHAVIOR

Obsessive-compulsive behavior is a psychological disorder in which the person becomes ruled by impulses, phobias, or preoccupations that compel him or her to repeat certain actions or sequences of actions, such as counting trees or washing the hands a thousand times a day. Sufferers, who are often highly intelligent, know their behavior is irrational but become exceedingly anxious if, for example, they miss counting a tree. Such behavior is agonizing for the person and family concerned, and sometimes results in suicide. Consult your doctor, who will likely refer you for psychological help.

Treatment

Behavioral therapy;
counseling; hypnotherapy;
psychotherapy.

OSTEOARTHRITIS

*A gradual degeneration of one or
more joints, osteoarthritis is
characterized by the knobby joints
often seen on fingers of afflicted
people. Osteoarthritis causes
increasing stiffness, sometimes
resulting in limited movement of
the affected joint or joints, and
pain, which is often worse at night.*

Treatment

Acupressure; acupuncture;
Alexander technique;
aromatherapy; auricular
therapy; Bach flower
remedies; biochemic tissue
salts therapy; chiropractic;
cymatic therapy; diet therapy
(especially if the sufferer is
overweight); herbal medicine;
homeopathy; hydrotherapy;
hypnotherapy; massage;
naturopathy; osteopathy;
physiotherapy; psychotherapy;
reflexology; sound therapy;
Tai Chi Ch'uan therapy; yoga.

OSTEOPOROSIS

*A thinning and weakening of the
bones, osteoporosis is more
common in elderly people, and
more common in women than
men. It gives rise to the loss of
height common in old age, and
can cause muscle spasms and
spontaneous fractures.*

Treatment

Diet therapy; homeopathy;
naturopathy; physiotherapy;
yoga.

PAIN

*Pain is the body's cry for help, a
warning that something,
somewhere is not as it should be.
It may be experienced as localized
pain, an immediately identifiable
specific area; or as referred pain,
in which the source of the pain is
remote, situated elsewhere. Pain
may stem from a physical,
emotional, psychological, or
spiritual source. Wherever it is,
whatever form it takes, pain
needs professional diagnostic help.
The following complementary
therapies offer pain relief.*

Treatment
Acupressure; acupuncture;
aromatherapy; auricular
therapy; autosuggestion
therapy; biochemic tissue salts
therapy; flotation therapy;
herbal medicine; massage;
visualization therapy.

PANIC ATTACKS

*A panic attack is a sudden,
overpowering sense of fear or
terror, an acute anxiety attack
that may arise from a physical,
emotional, or psychological
disturbance, shock, or trauma. A
terrifying condition, it can result
in hyperventilation
(overbreathing) and even loss of
consciousness. Professional help is
needed.*

Treatment
Acupuncture; Alexander
technique; aromatherapy; art
therapy; auricular therapy;
autosuggestion therapy;
autogenic training therapy;
Bach flower remedies;
behavioral therapy; biochemic
tissue salts; biofeedback;
counseling; dance therapy;

diet therapy; herbal medicine;
homeopathy; hydrotherapy;
hypnotherapy; massage;
meditation; megavitamin
therapy; music therapy;
naturopathy; yoga.

PEPTIC ULCERS

See Ulcers

PERIOD PROBLEMS

See Menopausal Problems,
Menstrual Problems,
Premenstrual Tension

PERSPIRING

See Sweating (Perspiring)

PHOBIAS

See Agoraphobia and
Claustrophobia

*Usually described, somewhat
unsympathetically, as irrational
fear, phobias often stem from a
frightening experience, such as*

being shut in a cupboard in childhood or stepping on a snake's nest. Common phobias include fear of animals, fear of germs, fear of insects, and fear of open or confined spaces. Symptoms may include dizziness, depression, fainting, nausea, vomiting, perspiring, and being unable to make a move for leisure or work. Phobias can be agonizing and may require professional help.

Treatment
Acupressure; aromatherapy; art therapy; autosuggestion therapy; Bach flower remedies; behavioral therapy; breathing for relaxation therapy; counseling; dance therapy; herbal medicine; homeopathy; hypnotherapy; meditation; music therapy; psychotherapy; reflexology; visualization therapy.

PIMPLES

Pimples may have physical causes, including overindulgence in the wrong kind of food, and emotional or psychological

disturbance, such as experiencing a shock or trauma.

Treatment
Aromatherapy; biochemic tissue salts therapy; diet therapy; herbal medicine; homeopathy; megavitamin therapy; naturopathy; physiotherapy.

POSTNATAL DEPRESSION

See Special Needs section, page 218

PREGNANCY

See Special Needs section, page 211

PREMENSTRUAL SYNDROME

Most women experience premenstrual syndrome at some time during their years of menstruation. Symptoms range from mild to severe and may include anxiety attacks, cramps, *cravings, depression, fluid retention, headaches, mood swings, and vertigo.*

Treatment
Acupuncture; aromatherapy; Bach flower remedies; breathing for relaxation therapy; diet therapy; herbal medicine; chiropractic or osteopathic spinal manipulation; homeopathy; massage; megavitamin therapy; naturopathy; physiotherapy; yoga.

PRICKLY HEAT RASH

See Heat Rash

PROLAPSE

Prolapse, a protruding or displaced organ, is most commonly used to describe the downward displacement of the rectum, a piece of bowel protruding through the anus, or prolapse of the uterus, which is common in women who have had several children. Consult your doctor or gynecologist.

Treatment
Acupressure; naturopathy.

PROSTATE PROBLEMS

Problems of the prostate, which affect men only, may consist of an enlarged prostate gland or inflammation and swelling of the prostate caused by infection. Symptoms include fever, an increased desire to urinate, and painful orgasm. Cancer must always be considered, so consult your doctor.

Treatment
Acupuncture; biochemic tissue salts therapy; breathing for relaxation therapy; diet therapy; herbal medicine; hydrotherapy (especially sitz baths and compresses); physiotherapy.

PSORIASIS

A distressing and chronic skin condition, psoriasis is commonly seen on the elbows and behind the knees but may affect all parts of

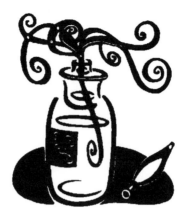

the body. It is recognized by its reddish patches with silvery, flaky scaling. It is not infectious, and the cause, despite many theories, remains unknown.

Treatment

Aromatherapy; Bach flower remedies; diet therapy; osteopathic spinal manipulation (to help treat constipation, which is considered to be a contributory factor); herbal medicine; homeopathy; hydrotherapy (especially alternate hot and cold showers); physiotherapy.

PSYCHOSOMATIC ILLNESSES

The expression, "It's all in the mind" sums up psychosomatic illnesses, with the reservation that what may start in the mind can impact the body, giving rise to serious ill health.

When an illness is primarily caused by psychosomatic factors—and doctors believe countless illnesses fall in this category—both the illness and the underlying emotional or psychological disturbance need treatment. What should be understood is that a psychosomatic illness is not an imaginary illness—on the contrary, it is as real as an illness with a physical origin.

Treatment
Autosuggestion therapy; Bach
flower remedies; behavioral
therapy; counseling; dance
therapy; hypnotherapy;
psychotherapy.

RASHES

See individual skin disorders
and childhood infections

RHEUMATISM

*Rheumatism is actually several
disorders, from mild to acute, that
cause pain in bones, muscles, and
joints. Consult your doctor.*

Treatment
Acupuncture; cymatic therapy;
diet therapy; herbal medicine;
homeopathy; hydrotherapy;
massage; reflexology; sound
therapy; yoga.

RHEUMATOID ARTHRITIS

*Rheumatoid arthritis is a chronic
inflammatory disease that causes*

*redness, swelling, tenderness, and
occasionally deformity of the joints.*

Treatment
Acupressure; acupuncture;
Alexander technique;
aromatherapy; auricular
therapy; Bach flower
remedies; biochemic tissue
salts therapy; chiropractic;
cymatic therapy; diet therapy
(especially if the sufferer is
overweight); herbal medicine;
homeopathy; hydrotherapy;
hypnotherapy; massage;
naturopathy; osteopathy;
physiotherapy; psychotherapy;
reflexology; sound therapy;
Tai Chi Ch'uan therapy; yoga.

RINGING IN THE EARS (TINNITUS)

*This intensely distressing problem
is also described as a roaring in
the ears. The persistent "noises"
in the head can have a
devastating effect on the sufferer
and often give rise to other
symptoms, such as depression and
a feeling of being trapped.
Consult your doctor.*

Treatment
Acupressure; acupuncture;
homeopathy.

SCALDS

See Burns and Scalds

SCHIZOPHRENIA

*One of the most common and
serious forms of mental illness,
schizophrenia is characterized by
abnormal, bizarre behavior,
including withdrawal from reality
and, possibly, delusions and
hallucinations. The exact cause is
not yet known, but hereditary
factors are thought to be
significant. The illness is
sometimes triggered by a
traumatic event, such as the
breakup of a romantic
relationship. Consult your doctor.*

Treatment
Breathing for relaxation
therapy; diet therapy;
counseling; chiropractic and
osteopathic spinal
manipulation; music therapy;
physiotherapy; psychotherapy.

SCIATICA

See also Back Pain

*Sciatica refers to pain along the
sciatic nerve, which runs down
the back of each thigh. Consult
your doctor.*

Treatment
Acupressure; acupuncture;
Alexander technique; auricular
therapy; autogenic training
therapy; biochemic tissue salts
therapy; chiropractic; cymatic
therapy; electrotherapy;
hydrotherapy; hypnotherapy;
kinesiology; massage;
osteopathy; reflexology; sound
therapy; Tai Chi Ch'uan
therapy; yoga.

SEIZURES

See Epilepsy

SEXUAL PROBLEMS

See Special Needs section,
page 221

SHINGLES

An acute viral infection of a nerve root that causes intense tingling pain and blisters in the skin directly associated with the nerve. Although the virus that causes shingles is identical to the virus that causes chicken pox, it is very rare for children with chicken pox to infect an adult with shingles. An adult with shingles, however, can infect a child with chicken pox. Consult your doctor.

Treatment
Acupuncture; aromatherapy; homeopathy; naturopathy.

SHOCK AND TRAUMA

Typical symptoms of a person in shock and trauma (the more severe form) are shallow breathing, coldness, dilated pupils, feeble but rapid pulse, nausea, dizziness, fatigue, headache, pallor, shivering, trembling, and weakness. Anxiety and panic attacks, nightmares, and sleeplessness may follow both conditions. Having received the appropriate emergency treatment, you may find the following complementary therapies helpful for easing remaining stress and tension.

Treatment
Acupuncture; Alexander
technique; aromatherapy; art
therapy; autogenic training
therapy; autosuggestion
therapy; Bach flower remedies
(the rescue remedy);
behavioral therapy;
bioenergetics; breathing for
relaxation therapy; cymatic
therapy; diet therapy; herbal
medicine; homeopathy;
hydrotherapy; hypnotherapy;
massage; meditation; music
therapy; reflexology; Rogerian
therapy; Tai Chi Ch'uan
therapy; visualization therapy;
yoga.

SINUSITIS

*An inflammation of the mucous
membrane lining of the sinuses
that connect with the nose,
sinusitis can be caused by an
allergic reaction, cold, or upper
respiratory tract infection. The
nose may feel plugged and have a
mucous discharge. Other symptoms
may include headache, and pain
behind the cheeks and eyes.*

Treatment
Acupuncture; aromatherapy;
herbal medicine; homeopathy;
massage; reflexology.

SKIN COMPLAINTS AND RASHES

See individual skin disorders
and childhood infections

SLEEP DISORDERS

See also Insomnia

*Sleep disorders may result from
physical, emotional, psychological,
or spiritual problems. They are
particularly common after shock
and trauma or changes in
routine, such as being away from
home or being in the hospital.
Treatment depends on whether it
is a short- or long-term problem.*

Treatment
Acupuncture; aromatherapy;
autogenic training therapy;
behavioral therapy;
biofeedback therapy;
breathing and relaxation
therapy; counseling; diet

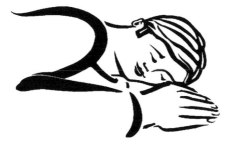

therapy; flotation therapy;
herbal medicine; homeopathy;
hydrotherapy; hypnotherapy;
massage; meditation;
naturopathy; physiotherapy;
psychotherapy; yoga.

SLIPPED DISC

*Slipped disc refers to a vertebral
disc that has become slightly
displaced and presses on a nerve,
causing agonizing pain. Common
causes are the making of sudden
abrupt movements, such as lifting
a heavy object, and whiplash
resulting from a car crash or
sports injury. See your doctor.*

Treatment
Acupressure; acupuncture;
chiropractic; cymatic therapy;
osteopathy.

SMOKING ADDICTION

*The following therapies are said
to help a smoker break with this
dangerous and possibly
life-threatening habit.*

Treatment
Acupuncture; auricular
therapy; autogenic training
therapy; autosuggestion
therapy; Bach flower
remedies; behavioral therapy;
counseling; flotation therapy;
homeopathy; hypnotherapy;
megavitamin therapy;
naturopathy; psychotherapy;
yoga.

SNEEZING

*Sneezing may provide relief in
moderation but is distressing when*

it happens all the time, as in certain allergic reactions such as hay fever.

Treatment
Aromatherapy; herbal medicine; naturopathy.

A cold sponge pressed against the face sometimes helps.

SNORING

Snoring usually occurs when the person is sleeping on the back with his or her mouth open, and it often ceases when the person turns onto the side or has the nostrils pinched together and chin lifted upward by a partner.

Treatment
Alexander technique; diet therapy; hypnotherapy; osteopathy; yoga.

SORE THROAT

See Laryngitis, Tonsillitis and Adenitis

SPORTS INJURIES

Sports injuries include back strains, concussion, pulled ligaments, torn tendons, strained muscles, sprains, bone fractures, and whiplash. See your doctor.

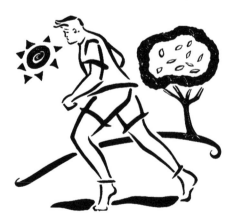

Treatment

Acupressure; acupuncture; Alexander technique; aromatherapy; autogenic training therapy; chiropractic; cymatic therapy; diet therapy; electrotherapy; homeopathy; hydrotherapy; hypnotherapy; massage; osteopathy; physiotherapy; reflexology; Shiatsu; sound therapy; Tai Chi Ch'uan therapy; yoga.

STAMMERING

Distressing, frustrating, and often embarrassing, stammering— halting, faltering, and hesitant speech—is usually due to spasm or incoordination of muscles. It may have an emotional and psychological cause as well as a physical one.

Treatment

Acupressure; Bach flower remedies; counseling; hypno- therapy; psychotherapy; yoga.

STINGS

See Insect Bites and Stings

STRESS

Although this term is often only associated with mental stress, it applies to physical and emotional stress, too—in other words, stress is the result of anything that disturbs the natural balance, physical, emotional, or mental. Practically every known ailment and disease could be listed here as being aggravated or caused by stress.

Treatment

Acupuncture; Alexander technique; aromatherapy; art therapy; autogenic training therapy; autosuggestion therapy; ayurvedic medicine; behavioral therapy; Bach flower remedies; bioenergetics; breathing for relaxation therapy; cymatic therapy; dance therapy; diet therapy; flotation therapy; herbal medicine; homeopathy; hydrotherapy; hypnotherapy; massage; meditation; music therapy; naturopathy; reflex- ology; Rogerian therapy; Shiatsu; Tai Chi Ch'uan therapy; visualization therapy; yoga.

STYES

Styes are small, pus-filled abscesses caused by inflammation of a gland at the edge of the eyelid.

Treatment
Herbal medicine; naturopathy.

SUNBURN

Painful reddening and peeling of the skin caused by prolonged exposure to the sun or heat haze. Pale-skinned people are most at risk. Too much sun exposure can cause skin cancer; prevention is easier than cure.

Treatment
Herbal medicine; naturopathy.

SWEATING (PERSPIRING)

Physical exertion, emotional and psychological issues, stress, obesity, and pain can all cause sweating to excess. If sweat remains on moist skin, it attracts bacteria and produces an unpleasant odor. Hot sweats may be the result of illness.

Cold sweats are usually brought about by excessive nervousness, anxiety, and panic attacks.

Treatment
Acupressure; aromatherapy; homeopathy; naturopathy.

TEETH GRINDING

Habitual teeth grinding can actually wear down the tooth enamel. This condition may stem from anxiety, pain, tension, or stress, and it usually occurs when the person is asleep. First consult a dentist, who may want to create a mouth guard for you.

Treatment
Acupressure; acupuncture; breathing for relaxation therapy; counseling; hypnotherapy; massage; osteopathy; psychotherapy.

TEMPER TANTRUMS

Common in adults as well as toddlers and children, temper tantrums are uncontrollable displays of rage: crying, shrieking, thumping, and lying on the floor kicking the feet in the air. It is best not to interrupt an adult during a tantrum; he or she is not in a mood to be reasoned with, and the sheer force of the tantrum may render a person blind and deaf to all entreaties. The underlying cause—for example, frustration, grief, or despair—needs professional investigation.

Treatment
Bach flower remedies; behavioral therapy; counseling; herbal medicine; hypnotherapy; naturopathy; psychotherapy.

TENNIS ELBOW

See also Bursitis

Tennis elbow is caused by frequent jarring that produces stiffness and pain in the elbow; it is common in carpetlayers, for example, because of repetitive hammering. It is a repetitive stress injury to the muscle on the outer side of the elbow joint or an inflammation of the bursa lying beneath the muscle.

Treatment
Aromatherapy; herbal medicine; homeopathy; hydrotherapy; massage; naturopathy; physiotherapy; osteopathy.

TENSION

Caused by physical, emotional, or mental strain, tension gives rise to many symptoms, including headaches, backache, cramps, depression, nervous disorders, temper tantrums, and other outbursts of anger and violence. The underlying cause needs investigating and alleviating.

Treatment
Acupuncture; Alexander technique; aromatherapy; art therapy; auricular therapy; autogenic training therapy; autosuggestion therapy; ayurvedic medicine; behavioral therapy; bioenergetics; biofeedback therapy; breathing for relaxation therapy, cymatic therapy; diet therapy; flotation therapy; Gestalt therapy; homeopathy; hydrotherapy; hypnotherapy;

kinesiology; meditation; music therapy; naturopathy; reflexology; Rogerian therapy; Shiatsu; Tai Chi Ch'uan therapy; visualization therapy; yoga.

THROAT PROBLEMS

See also Laryngitis, Tonsillitis and Adenitis

Problems of the throat are typically accompanied by pain and difficulty in talking and swallowing. Consult your family doctor.

Treatment
Diet therapy; herbal medicine (gargling); homeopathy; hydrotherapy (especially compresses); naturopathy; Shiatsu.

THRUSH (CANDIDA)

An infection caused by a fungus, thrush can affect the mouth, anus, vagina, nails, and skin. Symptoms include creamy white patches and the skin may also be inflamed with a red rash. Vaginal discharge may be present, and sexual intercourse may be painful. Consult your doctor.

Treatment
Aromatherapy; biochemic tissue salts therapy; diet therapy; herbal medicine; homeopathy; naturopathy.

THYROID DISORDERS

The thyroid gland, at the base of the neck, regulates the body's metabolism. Any disorder affecting this needs medical attention. Symptoms of thyroid disorder include the feeling that everything is spinning or is on fast-forward or rewind.

Treatment
Acupuncture; diet therapy; herbal medicine; homeopathy; reflexology.

TINNITUS

See Ringing in the Ears (Tinnitus)

TIREDNESS

See Fatigue (Exhaustion)

TONSILLITIS AND ADENITIS

Symptoms of inflammation and infection of tonsils and adenoids include a chill, fever, red and swollen sore throat, and difficulty in swallowing. With persistent inflammations, consult a doctor.

Treatment
Diet therapy; herbal medicine (gargling); homeopathy; hydrotherapy (especially compresses); naturopathy; physiotherapy.

TOOTH AND GUM PROBLEMS

Consult your dentist at once about any problems with the teeth or gums. The following may be helpful.

Treatment
Acupuncture; herbal medicine; homeopathy; hypnotherapy; Shiatsu.

ULCERS

There are several kinds of ulcers: duodenal and gastric, leg, mouth, peptic, and varicose. Consult your doctor.

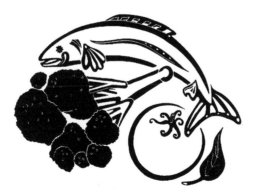

Treatment
Duodenal and Gastric
Acupuncture; autogenic
training therapy; diet therapy;
homeopathy; hydrotherapy
(especially pain-relieving
compresses); naturopathy;
physiotherapy.

Leg
Acupuncture; Alexander
technique; diet therapy;
herbal medicine; homeopathy;
naturopathy.

Mouth
Diet therapy; herbal medicine;
homeopathy; naturopathy.

Peptic
Acupuncture; Alexander
technique; autogenic training
therapy; diet therapy (Hay);
herbal medicine; homeopathy;
hydrotherapy (especially
pain-relieving compresses);
naturopathy; physiotherapy;
yoga.

Varicose
Alexander technique; diet
therapy; herbal medicine;
naturopathy; physiotherapy.

URINARY PROBLEMS

See Cystitis, Incontinence,
Kidney Stones, Prostate
Problems

VAGINAL DISORDERS

See Thrush, Vaginitis

VAGINITIS

*Vaginitis is inflammation and
acute irritation of the vagina.
Symptoms include intense
itchiness, redness, vaginal
discharge, odor, painful sexual
intercourse, swelling, and
tenderness. Consult your doctor.*

Treatment
Aromatherapy; biochemic
tissue salts therapy; diet
therapy; herbal medicine;
homeopathy.

VARICOSE VEINS

Common in people whose jobs entail standing for prolonged periods, varicose veins are unsightly, dilated, twisted veins often seen on the legs. Symptoms can include muscle cramps, swelling of the ankles, and tired legs. Consult your doctor.

Treatment
Alexander technique; diet therapy; exercise therapy; naturopathy; osteopathy; physiotherapy; yoga.

VERTIGO

Vertigo does not apply only to heights. The word is used to describe any kind of unsteadiness, such as dizziness, giddiness, or a feeling of falling or spinning. There are many possible physical, emotional, and mental causes. The distress experienced by the sufferer may be severe and can result in a desire not to go anywhere, even across a room in company, lest the affliction should suddenly strike. The underlying cause needs patient investigation.

Treatment
Acupressure; acupuncture; behavioral therapy; breathing for relaxation therapy; counseling; hydrotherapy; hypnotherapy; psychotherapy.

VIRAL INFECTIONS

Research has identified many viruses that are responsible for a wide range of illnesses, from the common cold to hepatitis and smallpox. Drugs and antibiotics have little impact on viruses; conventional medications usually treat only the symptoms of viral infections.

Treatment
Herbal medicine; homeopathy; megavitamin therapy; naturopathy.

VITAMIN DEFICIENCY

Most people who have a reasonably well-balanced diet are thought to receive sufficient vitamins. Unfortunately, many people do not have a reasonably well-balanced diet. Deficiencies also occur during some acute illnesses, such as jaundice, or after stomach or other surgery. Pregnant women and breast-feeding mothers also sometimes benefit from vitamin supplements.

Treatment
Diet therapy; kinesiology; megavitamin therapy.

WARTS

Warts are usually caused by a virus. Characterized by growths on the surface of the skin, they vary in size and shape but are usually small. They do not normally cause symptoms unless they are on the soles of the feet, in which case friction can cause discomfort.

Treatment
Acupuncture; aromatherapy; diet therapy; hypnotherapy; naturopathy.

WASP STINGS

See Insect Bites and Stings

WATER RETENTION

See Fluid Retention (Edema)

WEIGHT LOSS

The following complementary therapies are said to be an aid to losing weight and for people who have a health-threatening obesity problem.

Treatment
Acupuncture; breathing for relaxation therapy; diet therapy; electrotherapy (ENS); homeopathy; hydrotherapy (especially sauna and hot and cold showers to stimulate circulation); naturopathy; physiotherapy; yoga.

Counseling and psychotherapy may be necessary if the person concerned is deeply upset or worried about being obese.

WHEEZING

Wheezing refers to the harsh-sounding breathing, accompanied by a whistling sound that is common to asthma, bronchitis, emphysema, and hay fever sufferers. With all these conditions, the cause may be physical, emotional, or psychological.

Treatment
Acupuncture; Alexander technique; aromatherapy; auricular therapy; Bach flower remedies; biochemic tissue salts therapy; bioenergetics; chiropractic; diet therapy; herbal medicine; homeopathy; hydrotherapy; massage; meditation; naturopathy; osteopathy; physiotherapy; reflexology; visualization therapy; yoga.

WHOOPING COUGH

An acute childhood infection of the bronchi and trachea, whooping cough is easily recognized by the paroxysmal coughing spasms that end in a long "crowing" sound. Even the mildest whooping cough can be extremely disturbing and uncomfortable. Consult your doctor.

Treatment
Chiropractic; diet therapy; herbal medicine; homeopathy; massage; hydrotherapy; naturopathy; osteopathy; physiotherapy.

WORMS

Worm infestation may be by hookworms, pinworms, roundworms, and tapeworms. Symptoms may include itchy anus, loss of vitality, tiredness, and weight loss. Consult your doctor to eliminate worms. The following therapies can help restore health.

Treatment
Diet therapy; herbal medicine; homeopathy; naturopathy.

PART THREE

COMPLEMENTARY THERAPIES FOR SPECIAL NEEDS

FAMILY MATTERS

NATURAL FAMILY PLANNING

Origins

Not so very long ago, there was nothing but natural family planning. Then various methods of contraception were devised, followed by the contraceptive pill. Natural family planning came back into favor when people became anxious about the possible side effects and long-term effects of using a drug, the pill, to convince the body that it was pregnant so that it could not conceive. Many people began to voice doubts that keeping the body permanently in a state of "hoax pregnancy," or "full production" to avoid actual production, was asking for trouble and might possibly lead to a wearing down of the

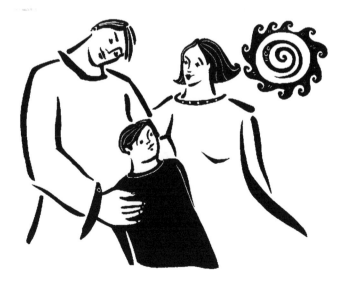

natural processes and to an inability to conceive a baby when one wanted to.

What it is   Natural family planning is not a therapy as such, but is nearly always included with other alternative and complementary therapies because it does not rely on artificial devices or drugs. Often called the *calendar* or *rhythm method,* it involves charting a woman's menstrual cycle, cervical changes, and basal body temperature in order to know when ovulation occurs—usually between twelve and sixteen days before the next period is due—and so to avoid the time when a women is most likely to conceive.

Charts and information about how to use natural family planning (sometimes referred to as the Billings method) can be obtained from your family doctor, gynecologist, or local community health center or women's clinic. See "Resources and Further Reading," page 264.

Two other methods that are considered natural but are not as reliable as charting a woman's menstrual cycle are *breastfeeding*—a mother is considered unlikely to conceive while she is breastfeeding her baby at least every two to four hours day and night—and *coitus interruptus*—the withdrawal of the penis before ejaculation. Some couples dislike this method because it mars the delight of sexual intercourse. Also, because semen may leak out before ejaculation or come in contact with the vagina after withdrawal, it is not considered an altogether effective family-planning method.

Artificial methods

Artificial birth-control methods include the condom, diaphragm, cervical cap, contraceptive pills, intrauterine device (IUD), spermicidal vaginal sponge, and morning-after pill.

IUDs, the pill, and morning-after pills are considered health threatening: IUDs can cause infection and heavy bleeding during menstruation; contraceptive pills increase the risk of breast cancer and blood clots and are considered unsuitable for women who smoke or who have existing health problems (family doctors or pharmacists can advise). In addition, some researchers say they may cause delays in wanted conceptions, and infertility. The morning-after pill, often referred to as the "abortion" pill, is considered inadvisable for long-term, routine use because it can have side effects, including nausea and painful spasms.

What doctors think

Some doctors regard anything but artificial devices and drugs as unreliable. Others believe that health, ethical, and religious considerations far outweigh the dangerous side effects and long-term effects of artificial devices and drugs, and that couples are well advised to persevere with natural family planning methods.

Warning

When using the natural family planning chart system, you may become pregnant if health problems or emotional stress alter the rhythm of menstruation and, therefore, the time of ovulation.

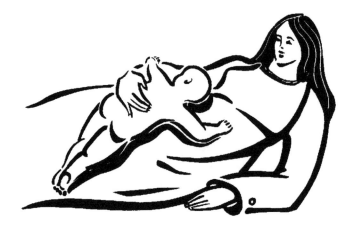

PREGNANCY

See also Childbirth

A healthy pregnancy

Many women are radiantly healthy during pregnancy; others experience common ailments, such as back pain, headaches, indigestion, morning sickness, and hemorrhoids. Morning sickness mainly affects the first three months of pregnancy. When seeking help, always mention that you are pregnant.

A healthful diet is essential at all stages of life, but is particularly important for women who are considering having a baby and who are pregnant.

Doctors advise against sexual intercourse during the first three months of pregnancy, and during the first six weeks after giving birth. Sexual intercourse during the latter stages of pregnancy sometimes causes contractions but is thought unlikely to induce labor.

Treatment   Alexander technique; aromatherapy; breathing
for relaxation therapy; herbal medicine; massage
(to ease back pain); meditation; naturopathy.
Osteopathy can be helpful for back pain caused
by a previous pregnancy. Herbal medicine,
homeopathy, and naturopathy are useful for
morning sickness.

Warning   It is important to consult your doctor or prenatal
clinic before beginning complementary therapies
or breathing and relaxation exercise programs.
The golden rules are never repeat anything that
causes you pain, and never push yourself beyond
what is comfortable.

CHILDBIRTH

**Current
Childbirth
Practices**   During the last two decades, there has been
much unrest about what have been called
"convenience births"—convenient, it has been
claimed, for the medical profession rather than
for the mother-to-be. Many people believe that
childbirth, a natural event, has been redefined by
the medical establishment and is now a very
sophisticated but unnatural event. Many
mothers-to-be are dismayed and overwhelmed to
find themselves lying in what feels like a cold,
clinical, surgical operating theater, attached to
fetal monitors and surrounded by frightening,
high-tech equipment. Many people are alarmed
by the increase in Cesarean births. Others
dispute the now-common practice of inducing
births—rupturing the bag of waters to start

labor—rather than waiting for the water to break naturally. Is this, it has been asked, really for the convenience of the medical staff?

Such criticisms are passionately contested by the medical profession: clinical surroundings are hygienic; the high-tech equipment is for the safety of mother-to-be and baby; births are induced and Cesareans performed only when it is considered necessary for the well-being of the mother and baby.

Many gynecologists and obstetricians have listened to these concerns, and many have made improvements and the best provision they can for mothers-to-be who insist on the minimum of medical intervention while they are bringing their baby into the world.

Natural childbirth

Natural childbirth, first coined by Dr. Grantly Dick-Read at the start of this century, aims for childbirth—in squatting, sitting, or standing positions—preferably without the use of pain-killing drugs. Instead, breathing and relaxation techniques are used to help mothers-to-be to counteract their fear of childbirth and to assist the process of labor and the birth. Midwives, counselors, and classes continue to teach a range of different natural childbirth methods.

Birth-without-violence techniques

Women have become more articulate, vocal, and mobilized about how they wish to give birth. A number have become devotees of sympathetic gynecologists, such as the French doctor Frederick Le Boyer with his birth-without-violence techniques. These techniques consist of soft lighting, soft voices, gentle handling, no slap on the baby's bottom, "bonding" time with the mother before the cutting of the umbilical cord, and the gentle immersion of the baby into warm water to soothe her or him after the struggle of being born.

Water births

Some women have become devotees of the French gynecologist Michel Odent, who pioneered the technique of giving birth in water—hydrotherapy—to ease labor pains.

Some modern maternity hospitals now offer tubs and pools for their mothers-to-be to give birth in water, and equipment for home births can be rented.

Natural treatment

Some women, alarmed by tales of the dangerous effects of some orthodox drugs on the development of the fetus and fearful of the still-discussed "thalidomide babies" tragedy, turn to Bach flower remedies, herbal medicine, and homeopathy for treatments during pregnancy.

Recommended complementary therapies for women who are pregnant or who wish to use natural childbirth are acupressure; acupuncture; aromatherapy; autogenic training therapy; Bach flower remedies; breathing for relaxation therapy; diet therapy (healthy living); herbal medicine; homeopathy; hypnotherapy (to help relaxation); massage (to ease lower back pain); meditation; naturopathy; yoga.

Warning

Always consult your doctor or prenatal clinic before commencing a complementary therapy.

POSTNATAL DEPRESSION

Postnatal depression, which may arise from a temporary hormonal imbalance after pregnancy and childbirth, ranges from mild to severe. It may also be attributed to or exacerbated by a natural reaction to the sudden and overwhelming responsibility of motherhood, hormonal changes, and the exhaustion that can result from caring for a newborn day and night, and perhaps other children and a husband, too! Consult your doctor or clinic.

According to the severity of the depression, the following complementary therapies may offer relief: acupuncture; Alexander technique; aromatherapy; autosuggestion therapy; autogenic training therapy; Bach flower remedies; breathing and relaxation therapy; counseling; diet therapy; herbal medicine; homeopathy; hydrotherapy; hypnotherapy; massage; meditation; megavitamin therapy; naturopathy; psychotherapy; yoga.

FAMILY HEALTH AND FITNESS

There has been much publicity recently concerning lack of exercise in children. Children today are less active than in past generations, and this will take its toll on their physical, emotional, and mental health, now and in the future. Street games, park games, sports, scouting activities, walks, swimming, cycling, and skating are being abandoned for video games and more and more television. An increase in diseases associated with an unfit body, such as heart disease and its related health problems, are mentioned on an almost daily basis.

The solution, of course, is exercise. Parents might begin by choosing a complementary therapy, such as breathing and relaxation exercises, to get themselves fit, and then set an example for their children to follow. The other family health concern is diet. No parent will go far wrong by their children if they abandon convenience foods for a healthful diet.

CHILDREN WITH PHYSICAL OR MENTAL DISABILITIES

The following complementary therapies are recommended for children who are in wheelchairs, are bedridden, or are long-term residents in hospitals or care centers: art therapy, massage, music therapy, hydrotherapy, and physiotherapy.

Autism   The autistic child appears to be completely withdrawn, lethargic, and living in a world of his

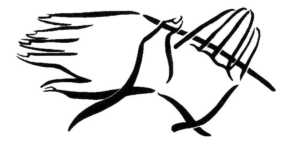

or her own. Emotional responses are rare, except occasional outbursts of rage.

The following complementary therapies have achieved some success: dance therapy, metamorphic technique, and music therapy.

Down's syndrome
The adult intelligence of those affected by Down's syndrome can be roughly equivalent to a three- to six-year-old child; they have very amiable, cheerful, affectionate, and lovable dispositions.

Metamorphic technique and music therapy are said to be useful complementary therapies.

Common Childhood Infections

See Chicken pox (page 163), Measles (page 183), Mumps (page 187), Whooping cough (page 209).

Sexuality

Enhancing Sex

The aromatherapy essential oils that are claimed to act as aphrodisiacs (stimulating sexual desire) when burned include: coriander, ginger, jasmine, neroli, patchouli, rose otto, sandalwood, vetiver, and ylang-ylang.

Other sex-enhancing therapies include herbal medicine (for example, ginseng in the form of tablets, teas, or tonics); massage (especially aromatherapy massage), naturopathy (remedies can be suggested by naturopaths, according to individual needs).

SEXUAL PROBLEMS

Most sexual disorders fall into four main categories: desire disorders, arousal disorders, orgasm disorders, and pain problems.

Desire disorders include deficient or absent sexual fantasies and desire, and sexual aversion, which is avoidance of sex. *Arousal disorders* affect both men and women, and may leave men unable to achieve or maintain an erection. *Orgasm disorders* include inhibited orgasm in both sexes, and premature or delayed ejaculation in males. *Pain disorders* include *dyspareunia,* which is genital pain before, during, or after sexual intercourse, and *vaginismus,* a painful condition in women that makes penetration impossible.

Other fairly common problems include dryness of the vagina, and injury, infection, inflammation, or ulceration of the female or male genitalia. Some orthodox drug treatments and some illnesses can affect sexual desire, performance, and satisfaction.

Common psychological problems affecting sexual intercourse include anxiety; depression; fear of failure to please or to be pleased or to satisfy or be satisfied or, as Woody Allen once put it, "fear of having the wrong kind of orgasm"; inhibition; stress; tension; tiredness; and, yes, headaches, possibly caused by *not* wanting sexual intercourse.

Couples experiencing serious and long-term sexual problems that are affecting them physically, emotionally, and mentally should consult their doctor or a therapist, preferably before the marriage or relationship is seriously threatened.

Treatment

Alternative therapies recommended for general sexual problems are Bach flower remedies, behavioral therapy, counseling, hypnotherapy, and psychotherapy.

Bach flower remedies recommended to help with sexual difficulties include centaury for people who feel they cannot say no; clematis for sexual lethargy and inactivity; crab apple for feeling that sex is shameful; heather for being selfish about one's sexual desires; honeysuckle for feeling romantic but sexually inadequate; and mimulus for fear of being overwhelmed by sexual urges.

The inability to get pleasure from sexual intercourse may, sooner or later, result in a reluctance to try, or complete abstinence. It may be due to a physical cause, such as painful sexual intercourse; the sexual inexperience of the couple, or a host of psychological problems stemming from negative attitudes toward sex. Suitable therapies include acupuncture, aromatherapy, Bach flower remedies, behavioral therapy, counseling, and psychotherapy.

The inability of a man to attain or maintain an erection during sexual intercourse can have physiological, emotional, or psychological causes. Suitable therapies include aromatherapy;

autogenic training therapy; behavioral therapy; chiropractic; counseling; diet therapy; hydrotherapy (especially hot and cold sitz baths); osteopathy; physiotherapy; and psychotherapy.

Infertility   The inability to have a child is considered to be on the increase; some claim it now affects one in six couples. The problem, which can have a multitude of causes, may stem from the female or male partner. Consult your doctor.

Suitable therapies include acupuncture, diet therapy, hydrotherapy, and naturopathy.

SPORTS INJURIES

The most common sports injuries are the following: back injuries; blisters; bursitis; cartilage damage; cramps; lacerations; bruised, pulled, whiplash, and torn ligaments; dislocations; muscle bruises and strains; sprains; "stitch" pain; tendon problems, including inflammation and rupture; repetitive stress injuries.

Treatment   Complementary therapies that are recommended for sports injuries include acupressure; acupuncture; Alexander technique; aromatherapy; autogenic training therapy; chiropractic; cymatic therapy; diet therapy; electrotherapy; homeopathy; hydrotherapy; hypnotherapy; massage; osteopathy; physiotherapy; reflexology; Shiatsu; sound therapy; Tai Chi Chu'an therapy; yoga.

The following complementary remedies are recommended for getting fit for sports activities:

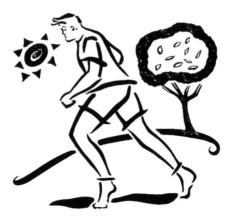

diet therapy (healthy living); breathing for relaxation therapy; hydrotherapy; massage (all kinds); meditation; physiotherapy; yoga.

Warning

Health checkups are important before taking up a new exercise regime or sport.

Never neglect discomfort or pain—it is the body's alarm system. Delays—and inappropriate treatment—can cause further damage and more serious long-term problems.

For serious discomfort, first consult your doctor or go to the nearest emergency room or urgent care center. Bone fractures, including stress fractures, are common sports injuries that need urgent medical attention. Dizziness, drowsiness, and nausea can indicate concussion.

APPENDIX

EASTERN RELIGIONS

So many complementary therapies stem from, and are based on, eastern religious disciplines that I think it important to include brief descriptions of the main eastern religions involved. Some people take up a new complementary therapy, and discover that they have also taken up a new religion.

All of these eastern religions differ fundamentally, both in belief and practice, from Christianity, the main religion of western countries and also practiced in many others. Some eastern religions require great discipline from their followers. People of sound mind will not be troubled by taking on new disciplines and responsibilities and may well grow in health and strength. For others, caution may be warranted.

BUDDHISM

Buddhists do not believe in a single god, the creator, but many Buddhists worship an array of gods—for example, the gods of kindness and wisdom—and many worship the Buddha as a god.

At the very heart of Buddhism is the belief that we should never cause harm to anybody or to any living thing. This is why many Buddhists are vegetarians.

At the heart of Buddhism is self-discipline aimed achieving detachment from the distractions of the world and inward peace. It

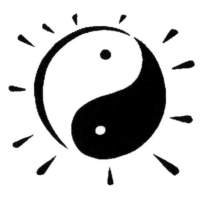

emphasizes compassion and the spreading of this peace. Through daily meditation, Buddhists hope to reach nirvana, the freedom from desire and the liberation from "becoming" things or selves. Buddhists believe in reincarnation—that each of us will be born again and again until we reach nirvana, when we will understand the Buddha's Four Noble Truths of the Noble Eightfold Path. The Four Noble Truths are

1. That human life is full of suffering.

2. That *we* create this suffering.

3. That if we hang on to pleasurable things— passing distractions and desires—at the expense of that which is eternal, spiritual—the collective good of all—suffering will continue.

4. That the Noble Eightfold Path is the way to tread, following in the footsteps of the Buddha, who surrendered a life of luxury to seek an answer to why people suffer.

The Noble Eightfold Path consists of

1. Right views—think positively, especially of the good in oneself, in others, and in creation.

2. Right thoughts—care for others and everything in creation.

3. Right speech—tell the truth and be gentle and kind with words.

4. Right action—do not kill, steal, or cause injury.

5. Right livelihood—do not cheat or harm anybody.

6. Right effort—practice and work hard to follow the Eightfold Path.

7. Right mindfulness—be aware of the consequences of thoughts and actions.

8. Right concentration—a calm, collected, peaceful state of mind will arise from following the Noble Eightfold Path.

The Buddha's Five Precepts, or rules for everyday living, are

1. Be kind, helpful, and sympathetic and do not harm or kill humans or any other living creature.

2. Do not steal, and be generous to those who are in need.

3. Never take more than you need.

4. Do not tell lies or say anything that is harmful.

5. Never act carelessly, thoughtlessly, or irresponsibly.

Hinduism

Hinduism has a rich variety of expressions that range from the worship of many gods, to the devotional worship of gods as expression of the One God, to a mysticism that suspects all religious images and seeks the absorption of the individual in the impersonal divine force, or World-Spirit (the *Brahman*).

Generally, Hindus believe in one divine force, which takes three main forms: Brahma, the creator, Vishnu, the preserver, and Shiva, the destroyer. It also has hundreds of other divine forms, such as Lakshmi, the goddess of wealth, and Ganesha, the god of good beginnings.

Hindus believe in reincarnation, and they teach that in the next life we will enjoy the good and bad results of how we have lived this life. Since all beings are considered part of the one God that permeates all forms of life, Hindus believe it is wrong to harm or kill other creatures, and they are vegetarians.

Hindus follow three ways, set out in the *Bhagavad Gita,* to achieve union with the Divine Force.

1. The way of knowledge, the study of ancient spiritual texts such as the *Vedas, Upanishads, The Ramayana,* and *The Mahabharata* to understand the deeper meaning of life and the universe.

2. The way of action, *yoga,* including body and mind spiritual practices, such as meditation.

3. The way of devotion, *bhakti,* love of God

through service—that is, caring for everybody
and everything in creation.

SHINTOISM

Considered to be the oldest Japanese religion,
Shintoism means "the Way of the Gods." It
developed in the sixth century and its scriptures
date from the eighth century. Shintoism focuses
on a way of purification and respectful
communion with the divinities and spirits of the
Japanese tradition. It is closely linked to nature
and to the seasons and the harvests.

TAOISM

Taoism is probably the oldest Chinese religion.
Tao means "the Way," and Taoists seek to follow
the Way—to achieve prosperity, longevity, and
immortality through virtuous living. Virtue can

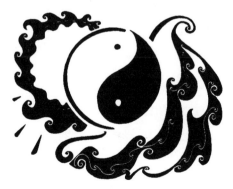

be understood as conformity to nature, both without and within humankind. Taoists believe we can ultimately live in complete harmony with the forces of the universe and in so doing, achieve immortality.

Some Taoists practice meditation in temples of beauty and tranquillity. They. believe the world is full of spirits, and use chants to call upon the spirits for healing and protection for themselves, their families, and the world. Some also believe in charms and magical formulae. Other Chinese religions are Zen Buddhism and Confucianism.

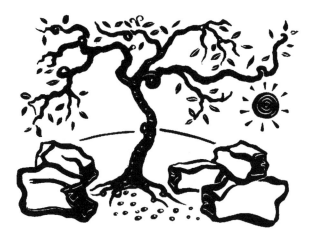

ZEN

Zen is the Japanese form of Buddhism. It is noted for a simple austerity, mysticism leading to personal tranquillity, and a focus on education and art. In addition to Buddhist disciplines and practices, it teaches that we need to get beyond the meaning of words to understand fully the meaning of life. For this reason, with the help of a master (a holy man), followers of Zen meditate on seemingly meaningless puzzles and parables to reach spiritual depths that lie beyond the surface of the mind and words. These lessons are intended to open the doors of perception into a world of wonder.

Resources and Further Reading

This section contains listings of organizations, books, retailers, and magazines organized by type of therapy. At the end of the chapter are general and health-issue specific resources. You may also find that your local yellow pages or classifieds will provide helpful local resources.

Acupressure

Acupressure Institute
1533 Shattuck Avenue
Berkeley CA 94709
(510) 845-1059

American Oriental Bodywork Association
6801 Jericho Turnpike
Syosset NY 11791
(516) 364-5533
Offers a professional membership association and program training.

Ohashi Institute
12 W 27th Street, Ninth Floor
New York NY 10001
(212) 684-4190, (800) 810-4190, fax: (212) 447-5819
Teaches Ohashiatsu, a method of bodywork offering a complete experience of self-development and healing. Ohashiatsu expands awareness of self and others through movement, meditation, and touch while relieving aches, tension, stress, and fatigue.

Ohashi International
Wallace Road
PO Box 505
Kinderhook NY 12106
Coordinates activities of Ohashiatsu schools in Europe. Coordinates and books speaking and teaching engagements for Ohashi.

Acupressure for Health: A Complete Self-Care Manual. Jacqueline Yong. London, England: Thorsons/HarperCollins, 1994.

Acupressure for Women. Catherine Bauer. Freedom, CA: Crossing Press, 1987.

Acupressure Way of Health: Jin Shin Do. Iona Marsaa Teeguarden. New York: Japan Publishers, 1978.

Reading the Body: Ohashi's Book of Oriental Diagnosis. Ohashi, with Tom Monte. New York: Penguin Arkana, 1991.

ACUPUNCTURE

American Association of Acupuncture and Oriental Medicine
433 Front Street
Catasauqua PA 18032
(610) 433-1433, fax: (610) 264-2768
Promotes public awareness of acupuncture and aims to gain legalization of acupuncture in all states, and insurance and Medicare coverage of acupuncture.

American College of Addictionology and Compulsive Disorders
5990 Bird Road
Miami FL 33153
(305) 661-3474, fax: (305) 538-2204

Offers national board certification in addiction and compulsive disorders treatment.

American Foundation of Traditional Chinese Medicine
505 Beach Street
San Francisco CA 94133
(415) 776-0502

American Medical Acupuncture Association
7535 Laurel Canyon Boulevard, Suite C
North Hollywood CA 91605

Center for Chinese Medicine
230 S Garfield Avenue
Monterey Park CA 91754

National Acupuncture Detoxification Association
3115 Broadway, Suite 51
New York NY 10027
(212) 993-0905

National Commission for the Certification of Acupuncturists
1424 16th Street NW, Suite 601
Washington DC 20036
(202) 232-1404

Traditional Acupuncture Foundation
American City Building, Suite 716
Columbia MD 31044

Acupuncture: How It Works, How It Cures. Peter Firebrace, B.Ac., MIROM and Sandra Hill, B.Ac, MIROM. New Canaan, CT: Keats Publishing, 1994.

Alexander Technique

North American Society of Teachers of the Alexander Technique
PO Box 517
Urbana IL 61801
(800) 473-0620
Provides membership services, public education, standards for certification of teachers, and teacher-training courses. Information and directory are available.

The Alexander Technique. Chris Stevens. New York: Charles E. Tuttle, 1987.

The Alexander Technique Workbook. Richard Brennan. Rockport, MA: Element Books, 1992.

Aromatherapy

Aroma Véra
5901 Rodeo Road
Los Angeles CA 90016-4312
(800) 669-9514, (310) 280-0407, fax: (310) 280-0395
Imports aromatherapy essential oils from around the world, conducts ongoing research and development in essential oils, and sells essential oils, aromatherapeutic skin and hair care, aromatic jewelry, and educational materials. An aromatherapy workbook, reference poster, and seminars are also available.

National Association for Holistic Aromatherapy
219 Carl Street
San Francisco CA 94117-3804
(415) 564-6785, fax: (415) 564-6799
Maintains high standards of aromatherapy education, establishes

professional and ethical standards of practice, provides public education, and publishes the quarterly, *Scentsitivity*.

National Association for Holistic Aromatherapy
PO Box 17622
Boulder CO 80308-0622
(415) 564-6785, fax: (415) 564-6799
Formulates standards of excellence and educates aromatherapy professionals and businesses.

Original Swiss Aromatics
PO Box 6842
San Rafael CA 94903
(415) 459-3998, fax: (415) 479-0614
Imports and distributes over a hundred medicinal-grade essential oils and aromatherapy products.

Pacific Institute of Aromatherapy
PO Box 6723
San Rafael CA 94903
(415) 479-9121, (415) 479-0119
Conducts research and offers education on essential oils.

Aromatherapy and the Mind. Julia Lawless. New York: Thorsons/HarperCollins, 1994.

The Complete Book of Essential Oils and Aromatherapy. Valerie Ann Worwood. San Rafael, CA: New World Library, 1991.

AUTOGENIC TRAINING THERAPY

British Association for Autogenic Training and Therapy
18 Holtsmere Close

Garston
Watford WD2 6NE
England
(011) 44-923-675501

Autogenic Therapy, Vol. 1. J. H. Schulz and W. Luthe. NY: Grune
and Stratton, 1969.

AYURVEDIC MEDICINES

American School of Ayurvedic Sciences
10025 NE Fourth Street
Bellevue WA 98004
(206) 453-8022

Ayurvedic Institute
1311 Menaul NE, Suite A
Albuquerque NM 87112
(505) 291-9698

Perfect Health. Deepak Chopra, M.D. New York: Harmony Books,
1990.

Prakruti: Your Ayurvedic Constitution. Dr. Robert E. Svoboda.
Albuquerque, NM: Geocom, 1989.

BACH FLOWER REMEDIES

Ellon USA
644 Merrick Road
Lynbrook NY 11563
(516) 593-2206

Flower Essence Society
PO Box 459
Nevada City CA 95959
(800) 548-0075, (916) 265-9163, fax: (916) 265-5467
Promotes plant research and empirical clinical research on the
therapeutic effects of flower essences, conducts seminars and
training and certification programs, and provides a communication
and referral network. Write or call for further information on their
research program, membership rates, discounts, class schedules,
newsletters, and other educational resources.

Pegasus Products
PO Box 228
Boulder CO 80306-0228
(800) 527-6104, (970) 667-3019, fax: (970) 667-3624
Produces and distributes a complete line of vibrational remedies
including flower essences, books, and tapes. Call or send for a catalog.

Perelandra
PO Box 3603
Warrenton VA 22186
(703) 937-2153, fax: (703) 937-3360
Operates a nature research center.

The Original Writings of Edward Bach. Judy Howard and John
Ransall. Essex, England: The C.W. Daniel Co., 1990.

Bach Flower Therapies. Mechthild Scheffer. Rochester, NY: Healing
Arts Press, 1988.

BIOCHEMIC TISSUE SALTS THERAPY

See also Homeopathy

Biochemic Handbook. Colin Lessell. London: Thorsons.

The Biochemic Tissue Salts Handbook. J. S. Goodwin. London: Thorsons.

BIOENERGETICS

Bioenergetics. Alexander Lowen. M.D. New York: Penguin Arkana, 1975.

BIOFEEDBACK THERAPY

Association for Applied Psychophysiology and Biofeedback
10200 West 44th Avenue, Suite 304
Wheatridge CO 80033
(303) 422-8436

Biofeedback Certification Institute of America
10200 West 44th Avenue, Suite 304
Wheatridge CO 80033
(303) 422-8436, (303) 420-2902

Biofeedback Society of America
U.C.M.C. c268
4200 E Ninth Avenue
Denver, CO 80262

Center for Applied Psychophysiology
Menninger Clinic
PO Box 829
Topeka KS 66601-0829
(913) 273-7500 Ext. 5375

Tools for Exploration
4460 Redwood Highway, Suite 2
San Rafael CA 94903
(415) 499-9050, fax: (415) 499-9047
Supplies health and consciousness technology products to the public.

BREATHING FOR RELAXATION THERAPY

Hendricks Institute
409 E Bijou Street
Colorado Springs CO 80903
(800) 688-0772, fax: (719) 632-0851
Offers personal and professional growth opportunities.

The Relaxation Response. Herbert Benson. New York: Outlet
Books, 1993.

CHIROPRACTIC

American Chiropractic Association
1701 Clarendon Boulevard
Arlington VA 22209
(800) 986-4636

Association for Network Chiropractic Spinal Analysis
PO Box 7682
Longmont CO 80501
(303) 678-8086

International Chiropractors Association
1110 N Glebe Road, Suite 1000
Arlington VA 22201
(703) 528-5000

World Chiropractic Alliance
2950 N Dobson Road, Suite 1
Chandler AZ 85224
(800) 347-1011

DANCE MOVEMENT THERAPY

American Dance Therapy Association
2000 Century Plaza, Suite 108
10632 Little Patuxent Parkway
Columbia MD 21044-3263
(410) 997-4040, fax: (410) 997-4048
Stimulates communication among dance/movement therapists and members of allied professions through publication of the *ADTA Newsletter* and the *American Journal of Dance Therapy*. ADTA holds an annual conference and supports formation of regional groups, conferences, seminars, and meetings.

DIET THERAPIES

Bristol Diet

American Dietetic Association
(800) 366-1655

Bristol Cancer Help Centre
Grove House
Cornwallis Grove, Clifton
Bristol BS8 4PG
England
helpline 44-117-974-3216; general inquiries 44-117-973-0500; fax: 44-117-923-9184
Provides complementary therapy, using a holistic approach, to people with cancer and those who care for them.

Gerson Therapy Diet

Gerson Institute
PO Box 430
Bonita CA 91908-0430
(619) 472-7450
Educates physicians and patients about alternative treatments for cancer, heart attack, and diabetes. Considers other options to surgery, chemotherapy, and similar medical procedures.

A Cancer Therapy: Results of Fifty Cases. Max Gerson. Del Mar CA: Totality Books, 1977.

Macrobiotic Diet Therapy

International Macrobiotic Shiatsu Society
1122 M Street
Eureka CA 95501-2442
(707) 445-2290, fax: (707) 445-2391
Acts as a forum for people interested in macrobiotics and Shiatsu.

Kushi Institute
PO Box 7
Beckett MA 01223
(413) 623-5741

Los Angeles East-West Center for Macrobiotic Studies
11215 Hannum Avenue
Culver City CA 90230
(310) 398-2228
Guides people in the use of food to establish health and happiness in accord with the laws of nature and the order of the universe. Offers personal consultations, cooking courses, workshops, and seminars on the philosophy and practical applications of the macrobiotic way of life.

Vega Study Center
1511 Robinson Street
Oroville CA 95965
(916) 533-4777, fax: (916) 533-4999
Emphasizes macrobiotic health education.

The Cancer Prevention Diet: Michio Kuchi's Nutritional Blueprint for the Relief and Prevention of Disease. Alex Jack, ed., and Michio Kushi. New York: Street Martin's Press, 1983.

Essential Oshawa. George Oshawa. Garden City Park, NY: Avery, 1994.

Mostly Macro. Lisa Turner. Rochester, NY: Healing Arts Press, 1995.

Nutritional Therapy

Natural Health **Magazine**
PO Box 1200
Brookline Village MA 02147
(617) 232-1000, fax: (617) 232-1572
Publishes a bimonthly magazine.

The Healing Foods: The Ultimate Authority on the Curative Power of Nutrition. Patricia Hausman and Judith Benn Hurley. New York: Avery, 1989.

A Consumer's Guide to Medicines in Food: Nutraceuticals that Help Prevent and Treat Physical and Emotional Illness. Ruth Weiner, M.S. New York: Crown, 1995.

Doctor, What Should I Eat? Isadore Rosenfeld, M.D. New York: Random House, 1995.

Native Nutrition: Eating According to Ancestral Wisdom. Ronal F. Schmid, N.D. Rochester, NY: Healing Arts Press, 1994.

Nutrition and the Mind. Gary Null, M.D. New York: Four Walls, Eight Windows, 1995.

A Consumer's Guide to Medicines in Food: Nutraceuticals that Help Prevent and Treat Physical and Emotional Illness. Ruth Weiner, M.S. New York: Crown, 1995.

Secrets of Natural Healing with Food. Nancy Appleton, Ph.D. Portland, OR: Rudra Press, 1995.

Super Healing Foods. Francis Sheridan Goulart. West Nyack, NY: Parker, 1995.

FASTING

Fasting Signs and Symptoms: A Clinical Guide. Trevor K. Salloum. East Palestine, OH: Buckeye Naturopathic Press, 1992.

The Hygienic System, Vol. III. Herbert M. Shelton. Chicago, IL: Natural Hygiene Press, 1971.

FELDENKRAIS METHOD

Feldenkrais Guild
PO Box 489
Albany OR 97321-0143
(800) 775-2118, fax: (503) 926-0572

Feldenkrais Resources
830 Bancroft Way, Suite 112
Berkeley CA 94710
(800) 765-1907, (510) 540-7600, fax: (510) 540-7683
Provides mail order sales of books and tapes of Feldenkrais and
other somatic fields.

*Awareness Through Movement: Health Exercises for Personal
Growth.* Moshe Feldenkrais. New York: Harper & Row, 1972.

The Potent Self: A Guide to Spontaneity. M. Feldenkrais and M.
Kimmey. San Francisco: Harper and Row, 1992.

Gestalt Therapy

Beyond the Hot Seat: Gestalt Approaches to Group. Bud Feder, ed.,
and Ruth Ronall. New York: Brunner/Mazel, Publishers, 1980.

Group Therapy

American Group Psychotherapy Association (AGPA)
25 E 21st Street, Sixth Floor
New York NY 10010
(212 477-2677, fax: (212) 977-6627
Advances knowledge of, research about, and training in group
psychotherapy for professionals and the public. AGPA provides a
network of peer support and advocates high standards and ethics
in group psychotherapy practice.

American Psychological Association (APA)
1200 Seventeenth Street, NW
Washington DC 20036

Association for Specialists in Group Work (ASGW)
599 Stevenson Avenue
Alexandria VA 22304

HELLERWORK THERAPY

The Body of Knowledge/Hellerwork
406 Berry Street
Mt. Shasta CA 96067
(916) 926-2500

HERBAL MEDICINE

American Association of Acupuncture and Oriental Medicine
433 Front Street
Catasauqua PA 18032
(610) 433-2448

American Association of Naturopathic Physicians
2366 Eastlake Avenue E, Suite 322
PO Box 20386
Seattle WA 98102

American Botanical Council
PO Box 201660
Austin TX 78720
(512) 331-8868, fax: (512)331-1924
Educates the public about beneficial herbs and medicinal plants through the journal *HerbalGram,* books, reprinted articles, and other educational materials.

American Herbalists Guild
PO Box 1683
Soquel CA 95073
(408) 464-2441, fax: (408) 464-2441, e-mail: Herbs@sensemedia.net
A nonprofit educational organization dedicated to the advancement of herbal medicine, and a peer-reviewe organization for professional herbalists who specialize in the medicinal use of plants. Membership includes discounts on all AHG resource materials and symposiums, and a subscription to the quarterly newesletter *The HerbaliStreet*. Resource materials include a comprehensive directory of herbal training programs, a recommended reading list, a code of ethics; an informed consent-full disclosure statement; and a membership directory.

Chinese Herbal Formulas for Women Only. Dr. Hong Yen Hsu and Douglas H. Easer. New Canaan, CT: Keats Publishing/Healing Arts Institute, 1982.

Earth Medicine, Earth Food: The Classic Guide to the Herbal Remedies and Wild Plants of the Native American Indians. Michael Weiner. New York: Fawcett, 1990.

A Handbook of Chinese Healing Herbs. Daniel Reid. Boston: Shambala, 1995.

Natural Healing and Herbs. Humbart Santillo, N.D. Prescott, AZ: Hohm Press, 1984, 1993.

HOMEOPATHY

British Institute of Homeopathy and College of Homeopathy
520 Washington Boulevard, Suite 423
Marina Del Rey CA 90292
(310) 306-5408, fax: (310) 827-5766

Provides in-depth training in homeopathy for a diploma or doctorate degrees.

Homeopathic Educational Services
2124 Kittredge Street
Berkeley CA 94704
(800) 359-9051, (510) 649-0294, fax: (510) 649-1955

International Foundation for Homeopathy
2366 Eastlake Avenue, Suite 325
Seattle WA 98102
(206) 324-8230

National Center for Homeopathy
801 N Fairfax Street, Suite 306
Alexandria VA 22314
(703) 548-7790, fax: (703) 548-7792

The Complete Homeopathic Handbook. Miranda Castro. New York: St. Martin's Press, 1991.

Homeopathic Medicine at Home. Maesimund B. Panos, M.D. and Jane Heimlich. New York: Jeremy P. Tarcher/Perigee, 1980.

Homeopathic Medicine for Children and Infants. Dana Ullman, M.P.H. New York: Jeremy P. Tarcher/Putnam, 1992.

Homeopathic Medicine for Mental Health. Insight Editions. Rochester, NY: Healing Arts Press, 1989.

Homeopathic Medicine for Women: An Alternative Approach to Gynecological Health Care. Trevor Smith, M.D. Rochester, VT: Healing Arts Press, 1989.

Homeopathy for Everyday Stress Problems. Insight Editions. Sussex, England: Insight Editions, 1993.

The Women's Guide to Homeopathy. Andrew Lockie, M.D. and Nicole Geddes, M.D. New York: St. Martin's Press, 1994.

HYDROTHERAPY

American Association of Naturopathic Physicians
2366 Eastlake Avenue E, Suite 322
Seattle WA 98102

National College of Naturopathic Medicine
11231 Southeast Market Street
Portland OR 97216
(503) 255-4860

Natural Health Clinic
1307 North 45th Street, Suite 200
Seattle WA 98103
(206) 632-0354
Provides clinical training for students while providing quality health care to the public.

Uchee Pines Institute
30 Uchee Pines Road, Suite 75
Seale AL 36875
(205) 855-4764

Your Body's Many Cries for Water. F. Batmanghelidj, M.D. Falls Church, VA: Global Solutions, 1995.

Hypnotherapy

American Board of Hypnotherapy
16842 Von Karman Avenue, Suite 475
Irvine CA 92714-4950
(714) 261-6400, fax: (714) 251-4632
Provides professional hypnotherapists with certification and
registration by an international organization and offers ongoing
education for hypnotherapists through trainings, seminars, and
conferences. Members receive the *ABH Journal* and discounts on
trainings and books.

American Society of Clinical Hypnosis (ASCH)
2200 East Devon Avenue, Suite 291
Des Plaines IL 60018
(708) 297-3317

International Medical and Dental Hypnotherapy Association
4110 Edgeland, Suite 800
Royal Oak MI 48073-2285
(800) 257-5467, (810) 549-5594
Provides trained certified hypnotherapists who will work in
harmony with local health-care professionals to aid individuals in
dealing with specific medical challenges and procedures.

National Guild of Hypnotists
PO Box 308
Merrimack NH 03054
(603) 429-9438

IRIDOLOGY

Applied Iridology and Herbology. Donald Banner. Bi-World Publishers.

Iridology: A Complete Guide to Diagnosing Through the Iris and to Related Forms of Treatment. Farida Sharan. London: Thorsons, 1989.

Iridology. Dorothy Hall. UK: Angus and Robertson, 1980.

KINESIOLOGY

International College of Applied Kinesiology
PO Box 905
Lawrence KS 66044-0905
(913) 542-1801

MASSAGE

American Massage Therapy Association
820 Davis Street, Suite 100
Evanston IL 60201-4444
(708) 864-0123, fax: (708) 864-1178
Provides referrals for qualified massage therapists in any local area.

Associated Bodywork and Massage Professionals
28677 Buffalo Park Road
Evergreen CO 80439-7347
(303) 674-8478, fax: (303) 674-0859
Dedicated to educating the public about the benefits of massage and bodywork, promoting ethical practices throughout the bodywork and massage industry, and protecting the rights of practitioners.

Esalen Institute
Big Sur CA 93920
(408) 667-3000
Encourages work in the humanities and sciences that promotes
human values and potentials. Activities include public seminars,
residential work-study programs, invitational conferences, and
research.

International Association of Infant Massage
2350 Bowen Road
Elma NY 14059
(800) 248-5432, fax: (716) 652-1990
Promotes nurturing touch and communication through training,
education, and research so that parents, caregivers, and infants are
loved and respected.

Massage **magazine**
PO Box 1500
Davis CA 95617
(916) 757-6033, fax: (916) 757-6041
Massage educates and informs massage therapists and allied health
professionals about techniques, trends, and developments in the
field of massage bodywork. The magazine runs interviews and
profiles of innovative therapists, in-depth technique articles, news
briefs, and feature articles. *Massage* has an international readership
of 50,000.

MEDITATION

Association for Transpersonal Psychology
PO Box 4437
Stanford CA 94309
(415) 327-2066

Provides information through conferences, membership, and publications in the field of transpersonal psychology.

Cambridge Insight Meditation Center
331 Broadway
Cambridge MA 02139
(617)491-5070, fax: (617) 441-9038
CIMC is a nonprofit urban center for the practice of insight meditation *(vipassana)* offering an environment where the contemplative life can be developed and protected amidst the complexities of city living.

Insight Meditation Society
1230 Pleasant Street
Barre MA 01005
(508) 355-4378, fax: (508) 355-6398
IMS operates a silent meditation retreat center for the intensive practice of insight meditation *(vipassana)* in the Theravada tradition of the teachings of the Buddha.

Insight Meditation West
PO Box 909
Woodacre CA 94973
(415) 488-0164

Institute of Noetic Sciences
PO Box 909
Sausalito CA 94966
(415) 331-5650

Maharishi International University
1000 North Fourth Street
Fairfield IA 52556
(515) 472-5031

Mind-Body Clinic
New Deaconess Hospital
Harvard Medical School
185 Pilgrim Road
Cambridge MA 02215
(617) 632-9530

Mind/Body Health Sciences, Inc.
393 Dixon Road
Boulder CO 80302
(303) 440-8460; fax: (303) 440-7580
Write or call for a free copy of the *Circle of Healing* newsletter.

MEGAVITAMIN THERAPY

The Natural Health Guide to Antioxidants: Supplements to Fight Disease and Maintain Optimal Health. Nancy Bruning, with the editors of Natural Health. New York: Bantam, 1994.

MUSIC THERAPY

American Association of Music Therapy
PO Box 80012
Valley Forge PA 19484
(610) 265-4006, (610) 265-1011
Dedicated to improving the quality of life through the use of music in therapy, establishing standards of professional competence, implementing those standards through certification of individuals and approval of university curricula, promoting and disseminating research through professional publications, and fostering community awareness of and public education in music therapy.

The Chalice of Repose Project
Street Patrick's Hospital
554 West Broadway
Missoula MT 59806
(406) 542-0001 Ext. 2810, fax: (406) 728-2206
Serves the physical and spiritual needs of the dying with
prescriptive music; educates clinicians, health-care providers, and
the public about the possibility of a blessed death and the gift that
conscious dying can bring to the fullness of life; and integrates and
models these contemplative and clinical values in daily practice.

The Georgiana Organization
PO Box 2607
Westport CT 06880
(203)454-1221, fax: (203)454-3733
Encourages the practice of Auditory Integration Training (AIT),
which may be helpful to people with learning and behavioral
problems.

Institute for Music, Health and Education
PO Box 4179
Boulder CO 80306
(303) 443-8484, fax: (303) 443-0053
A nonprofit educational institute dedicated to the exploration of
the sonic arts in education and therapy for innovative students and
professionals. Workshops, a directory, and membership are available.

Music Therapy Center
251 W 51st Street
New York NY 10019

The Healing Energies of Music. Hal A. Lingerman. Wheaton, IL:
Quest Books, 1995.

Music: Physician for Times to Come. Don Campbell, ed. Wheaton, IL: Quest Books, 1991.

Sacred Sounds: Transformation Through Music and Words. Ted Andrews. St. Paul, MN: Llewellyn, 1994.

NATURAL FAMILY PLANNING

The Fertility Awareness Handbook. Barbara Kass-Annese, R.N., C.N.P. and Hal Danzer, M.D. Alameda, CA: Hunter House, 1992.

The Billings Method. Evelyn Billings, M.D. New York: Ballantine, 1983.

NATUROPATHY

American Association of Naturopathic Physicians
2366 Eastlake Avenue E, Suite 322
Seattle WA 98102
(206) 323-7610, fax: (206) 323-7612
Provides national support for licensed and license-eligible naturopathic physicians, and offers public education and referrals.

Bastyr University
1307 North 45th Street, Suite 200
Seattle WA 98103
(206) 632-0354

Canadian College of Naturopathic Medicine
60 Berl Avenue
Etobicoke, Ontario M87 3C7
Canada
(416) 251-5261

Institute for Natural Medicine
66 1/2 North State Street
Concord NH 03301-4330
(603) 225-8844
Seeks to change the emphasis of our health-care system from
disease management to health promotion and disease prevention
using the principles of natural medicine.

National College of Naturopathic Medicine
11231 SE Market Street
Portland OR 97216
(503) 255-4860

OSTEOPATHY

American Academy of Osteopaths
3500 De Pauw Boulevard, Suite 1080
Indianapolis IN 46268
(317) 879-1881, fax: (317) 879-0563
Teaches, explores, advocates, and advances the study and application
of total health-care management, emphasizing osteopathic principles,
palpatory diagnosis, and osteopathic manipulative treatment.

American Osteopathic Association
142 E Ontario Street
Chicago IL 60611
(312) 280-5800

PHYTOTHERAPY

American Botanical Council
PO Box 201660
Austin TX 78720

American Herb Association
PO Box 1673
Nevada City CA 95959
(916) 265-9552
An educational organization dedicated to increasing knowledge about medicinal herbs through the *AHD Quarterly*, a directory of herbal education, and a book list.

American Society for Physiotherapy (ASAP)
PO Box 3679
South Pasadena CA 91031
(818) 457-1742

Herb Research Foundation
1007 Pearl Street, Suite 200
Boulder CO 80302
(303) 449-2265, fax: (303) 449-7849
A nonprofit, member-supported research and educational organization dedicated to providing reliable scientific botanical data for its members, the public, and the media.

Healing Plants. Mannfried Pahlow. Hauppauge, NY: Barron's Educational Series, 1993.

POLARITY THERAPY

American Polarity Therapy Association
2888 Bluff Street, Suite 149
Boulder CO 80301
(303) 545-2080, fax: (303) 545-2161
Advances polarity therapy by developing educational and support materials, registering practitioners, hosting educational conferences, and publishing literature.

Polarity Wellness Center
10 Leonard Street, Suite A
New York NY 10013
(212) 334-8392

Polarity Therapy. Alan Siegel, M.Sc., N.D. Santa Rosa: Prism
Press/Atrium Publishers, 1987.

PRIMAL SCREAM THERAPY

The New Primal Scream: Primal Therapy Twenty Years On. Arthur
Janov. Wilmington, DE: Enterprise Publishing, 1991.

REBIRTHING THERAPY

Rebirthing: The Science of Enjoying It All of Your Life. James Leonard
and Richard Lant. Cincinnati, OH: Vivation Publishing, 1983.

REFLEXOLOGY

International Institute of Reflexology
PO Box 12642
St. Petersburg FL 33733-2642
(813) 343-4811, fax: (813) 381-2807
Teaches and certifies people on a professional level, and upgrades
the standards of reflexology on an international basis. Provides
referrals for a reflexologist in any local area.

Better Health with Foot Reflexology. Dwight Byers. St. Petersburg,
FL: Ingham Publishing, 1987.

Body Reflexology: Healing at Your Fingertips. Mildred Carter. New
York: Parker Publishing, 1986.

Hand and Foot Reflexology: A Self-Help Guide. Kevin Dunz and Barbara Dunz. New York: Simon and Schuster, 1987.

Hand Reflexology: Keys to Perfect Health. Mildred Carter. West Nyack, NY: Parker Publishing, 1975.

REICHIAN THERAPY

International Journal of Life Energy
PO Box 8900
Station B
Willowdale, Ontario M2K 2R6
Canada

Journal of Biodynamic Psychology
Copy Centre
50 George Street
London W1A
England

Radix
PO Box 97
Ojai CA 93023

Character Analysis. Wilhelm Reich. New York: Simon and Schuster, 1972.

The Function of the Orgasm. Wilhelm Reich. Noonday Press, 1971.

The Man Who Dreamed of Tomorrow: A Conceptual Biography of Wilhelm Reich. Edward W. Mann and Edward Hoffman. Los Angeles CA: J. P. Tarcher, 1980.

Rolfing

The Rolf Institute of Structural Integration
205 Canyon Boulevard
Boulder CO 80302
(800) 530-8875, (303) 449-5903, (303) 449-5978
Selects, trains, and certifies qualified practitioners; provides
continuing education; promotes research; and educates the public
on Rolfing Structural Integration.

Rolfing: The Integration of Human Structures. Ida P. Rolf. New
York: Harper and Row, 1977.

Stress Therapies

Awareness and Relaxation Training
c/o Stress Reduction Program
Santa Cruz Medical Clinic
2025 Soquel Avenue
Santa Cruz CA 95062
(408) 458-5842
Provides a stress reduction program promoting healthful living and
wellness, modeled after the mindfulness-based stress-reduction
work of Jon Kabat-Zinn, Ph.D., from the Umass Medical Center
and featured in Bill Moyers' series "Healing and the Mind." Helps
people develop a more positive relationship to stress in their work
environment and daily lives, and complements the medical
management of a wide range of medical disorders.

Center for Mindfulness in Medicine, Health Care, and Society
University of Massachusetts Medical Center
Worcester MA 01655-0267
(508) 856-2656, fax: (508) 856-1977

Stress Reduction Clinic
c/o Camino Healthcare
2500 Grant Road
Mountain View CA 94039
(415) 940-7070; (408) 223-4040
Provides an educational program promoting healthful living, wellness, and stress management in which participants learn and practice the tools of awareness and relaxation. The program complements the medical management of chronic pain and stress-related disorders.

The Relaxation Response. Herbert Benson. New York: Outlet Books, 1993.

T'AI CHI CHU'AN

School of T'ai Chi Chuan
5 E 17th Street, Fifth Floor
New York NY 10003
(212) 929-1981, (212) 727-1852

T'ai Chi Chu'an and I Ching: A Choreography of Body and Mind. Da Liu. Harper and Row, 1972, 1987.

THERAPEUTIC TOUCH

Therapeutic Touch. Janet Macrae. New York: Knopf, 1987.

TRAGERWORK

Trager Institute
33 Millwood
Mill Valley CA 94941
(415) 388-2688, fax: (415) 388-2710

Trains and certifies individuals in the practice of Trager psychophysical integration and Mentastics movement education.

Trager Mentastics: Movement as a Way to Agelessness. Milton Trager and Cathy Guadagno. New York: Station Hill Press, 1987.

YIN AND YANG THERAPY

See Macrobiotic Diet Therapy under Diet Therapies

YOGA

Yoga Journal
P.O. Box 469018
Escondido CA 92046-9018
(510) 841-9200

Acu-Yoga: The Acupressure Stress Management Book. Michael Reed Gach with Carolyn Marco. New York: Japan Publishers, 1981

The American Yoga Association Beginner's Manual. Alice Christiansen. New York: Simon and Schuster, 1987.

Living Yoga: A Comprehensive Guide for Daily Life. Georg Geuerstein and Stephan Bodian, with the staff of Yoga Journal. New York: Tarcher/Putnam, 1993.

Yoga for Body, Mind, and Breath: A Guide to Personal Reintegration. A. G. Mohan. Portland, OR: Rudra Press and International Association of Yoga Therapists, 1993.

Yoga for Common Ailments. Dr. Robin Monro, Dr. Nagarathna, and Dr. Nagendra. New York: Simon and Schuster, 1990.

Yoga for Pregnancy. Sandra Jordan. New York: St. Martin's, 1987.

GENERAL NATURAL AND COMPLEMENTARY HEALTH

World Research Foundation
15300 Ventura Boulevard, Suite 405
Sherman Oaks CA 91403
(818) 907-5483
Compiles medical and scientific research from around the world. For a search fee, the foundation will provide information on the most current treatments for a variety of health conditions.

African Holistic Health. Llaila O. Afrika. Brooklyn, NY: A and B Books, 1993.
Traditional nutritional, herbal, and other natural approaches to health.

Alternative Resources. Brett Jason Sinclair. West Nyack, NY: Parker, 1992.
A comprehensive directory and annotated guide to natural and alternative health resources.

Back to Eden. Jethro Kloss. Loma Linda, CA: Back to Eden Publishing, 1939, 1994.
The self-described classic "guide to herbal medicine, natural foods, and home remedies."

Choices in Healing: Integrating the Best of Conventional and Complementary Approaches to Cancer. Michael Lerner. Boston: MIT Press, 1994.
A comprehensive overview of therapies for cancer patients, including nutritional supplements, anticancer diets, Chinese medicine, bodywork therapies, psychotherapy, and other methods.

The Complete Book of Chinese Health and Healing. Daniel Reid.
Boston: Shambala, 1995.
An review of the traditional Chinese healing therapies, including
herbs and plants, acupressure, T'ai Chi, and the philosophy of yin
and yang.

Encyclopedia of Natural Medicine. Michael Murray, N.D. and
Joseph Pizzorno, N.D. Rocklin, CA: Prima Publishing, 1991.
A classic reference, which discusses the use of herbs, vitamins and
minerals, and nutritional treatments.

Healing and the Mind. Bill Moyers. New York: Doubleday, 1993.
Based on the PBS series. Explores the connection between physical
and mental well-being in interviews with a variety of natural and
alternative health researchers and practitioners.

Menopause Without Medicine. Revised third edition. Linda Ojeda,
Ph.D. Alameda, CA: Hunter House, 1995.
Natural approaches to treating menopausal symptoms, including
nutrition, vitamin and mineral supplements, herbs, exercise, and
phytotherapies.

Mind as Healer, Mind as Slayer. Kenneth R. Pelletier. New York:
Delta, 1972, 1992.
A classic exploration into the mind-body connection.

Natural Alternatives to Over-the-Counter and Prescription Drugs.
Michael T. Murray, N.D. New York: Morrow, 1994.
A comprehensive guide to alternatives to drugs, including
prescription drugs for chronic ailments and health conditions and
over-the-counter treatments for colds, arthritis, headaches, and
other common conditions.

Natural Health, Natural Medicine: A Comprehensive Manual for Wellness and Self-Care. Andrew Weil, M.D. New York: Houghton Mifflin, 1995.
Provides an introduction to the philosophy and practice of self-care and natural healing.

Nontoxic, Natural and Earthwise. Debra Lynn Dadd. New York: Tarcher/Putnam, 1990.
Natural and nontoxic alternatives to household cleaners and other common products. Includes recipes for homemade alternatives and listings of commercially available products and where to find them.

Women's Bodies, Women's Wisdom: Creating Physical and Emotional Health and Healing. Christiane Northrup, M.D. New York: Bantam, 1994.
A thorough review of women's medical issues, natural and self-care measures, and a discussion of the traditional medical approach to women's health. Northrup is a former president of the American Holistic Medical Association.

Hunter House
MENOPAUSE / WOMEN'S CANCERS

MENOPAUSE WITHOUT MEDICINE
by Linda Ojeda, Ph.D.   *New Third Edition*

The revised third edition of this bestselling book provides comprehensive guidelines on holistic, natural ways to prepare for menopause and treat common complaints. Topics include nutrition, exercise, herbs and vitamin supplements, and natural sources of estrogen. Debunks the myths of menopause and emphasizes the excitement and fulfillment the later years of life can bring. *As seen in* Time *magazine.*

304 pages ... 12 illus. ... Paperback $13.95 ... Hard cover $23.95

THE MENOPAUSE INDUSTRY: How the Medical Establishment Exploits Women *by* Sandra Coney

Sandra Coney's groundbreaking book destroys the myth that menopause is a disease. She examines the benefits and exposes the risks of many common interventions like HRT, mammography, and cervical screening, and she urges women to trust their bodies first.

> **"Read this book and become enraged! . . . Sandra Coney's balanced approach gives information and therefore power back to all midlife women."** — Susan Love, M.D., author of *Dr. Susan Love's Breast Book*

400 pages ... 32 illus. ... Paperback $14.95 ... Hard cover $24.95

NO LESS A WOMAN: Femininity, Sexuality, and Breast Cancer *by* Deborah Hobler Kahane, MSW

In *No Less A Woman* ten women describe how they coped with the changes in their bodies, their feelings, and their lives. Their stories offer vital information other women with breast cancer can use in their own lives.

> **"An invaluable resource for all women going through the diagnosis, treatment, or emotional aftermath of the disease."** — Harriet G. Lerner, author of *The Dance of Anger*

304 pages ... Paperback ... $14.95

WOMEN'S CANCERS: How to Prevent Them, How to Treat Them, How to Beat Them *by* Kerry McGinn & Pamela Haylock

Women's Cancers focuses specifically on the cancers that affect only women—breast, cervical, ovarian, and uterine cancer. It describes successful prevention, detection, and cancer treatments. Includes a chapter on successful natural therapies.

> **"WOMEN'S CANCERS is fully comprehensive . . . . Highly recommended."** — *Library Journal*

448 pages ... 54 illus. ... Paperback ... $16.95

Prices subject to change

ORDER FORM

10% DISCOUNT on orders of $50 or more —
20% DISCOUNT on orders of $150 or more —
30% DISCOUNT on orders of $500 or more —
On cost of books for fully prepaid orders

NAME

ADDRESS

CITY/STATE   ZIP/POSTAL CODE

PHONE   COUNTRY (outside U.S.A.)

TITLE	QTY	PRICE	TOTAL
From Acupressure to Zen (paperback)		@ $15.95	
From Acupressure to Zen (hard cover)		@ $25.95	
Special: **All 3 A-to-Z books** *(paperback)*		@ **$34.95**	
Please list other titles below:			
		@ $	
		@ $	
		@ $	
		@ $	
		@ $	
		@ $	
		@ $	
		@ $	

Shipping costs:
*First book: $2.50
($6.00 outside U.S.)
Each additional book:
$.75 ($3.00 outside
U.S.)
For UPS rates and
bulk orders call us at
(510) 865-5282*

TOTAL _____
Less discount @_____%   (_____)
TOTAL COST OF BOOKS _____
Calif. residents add sales tax _____
Shipping & handling _____
TOTAL ENCLOSED _____
Please pay in U.S. funds only

❏ Check   ❏ Money Order   ❏ Visa   ❏ M/C   ❏ Discover

Card # _____ Exp date _____

Signature _____

Complete and mail to:

Hunter House Inc., Publishers
PO Box 2914, Alameda CA 94501-0914
Orders: 1-800-266-5592
Phone (510) 865-5282 Fax (510) 865-4295

❏ Check here to receive our book catalog

FAZ 11/95